QUACKS, ROGUES
AND CHARLATANS

First published in Great Britain in 2015 by Little, Brown

Copyright © Royal College of Physicians

The moral right of the authors has been asserted.

All images from RCP collections unless otherwise indicated.

Designed by Emil Dacanay and Sian Rance, D.R. ink

A CIP catalogue record for this book is available from the British Library.

ISBN 978-1-4087-0626-8

Printed in Italy

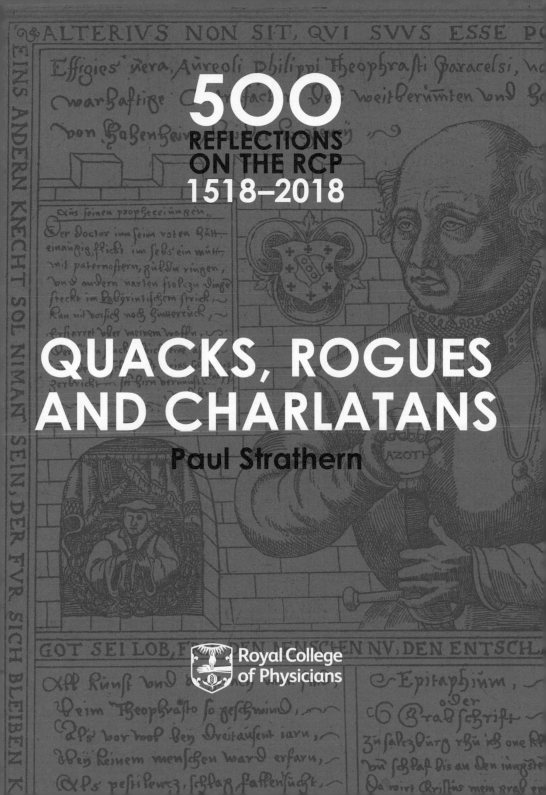

500
REFLECTIONS
ON THE RCP
1518–2018

QUACKS, ROGUES
AND CHARLATANS

Paul Strathern

**Royal College
of Physicians**

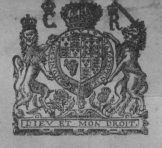

❧By the King.

¶ A Proclamation for the better ordering of those who repayre
to the Court, for their cure of the disease called the *Kings Euill.*

WHereas by the grace and blessing of God, the Kings and Queenes
of this Realme, by many ages past, haue had the happinesse, by their
sacred touch and inuocation of the Name of God, to cure those, who
are afflicted with the disease called the Kings Euill. And his now most
Excellent Maiestie, in no lesse measure then any of his Royall predecessors, hath had good successe herein, and in his most gracious and pious
disposition is as ready and willing, as any King or Queene of this
Realme euer was, in any thing to relieue the distresses and necessities
of his good Subiects; Yet in his Princely wisedome foreseeing that
in this, (as in all other things) order is to be obserued, and fit times are
fitly to be appointed for the performing of this great worke of charitie: His most excellent
Maiestie doth hereby publish and declare his Royall will & pleasure to bee, That whereas heretofore, the vsuall times of presenting such persons to his Maiesty for this purpose, were Easter and
Whitsuntide, That from henceforth the times shall bee Easter and Michaelmas, as times more
conuenient, both for the temperature of the season, and in respect of any contagion, which may happen in this neere accesse to his Maiesties sacred Person. And his Maiestie doth accordingly will
and command, That from the time of publishing this Proclamation, none presume to repayre to
his Maiesties Royall Court to bee healed of that disease, before the Feast of S. Michael now next
comming. And his Maiestie doeth further will and command, That all such as hereafter shall
come or repayre to the Court for this purpose, shall bring with them Certificates vnder the hands
of the Parson, Uicar, or Minister and Church-wardens of those seuerall parishes where they
dwell, and from whence they come, testifying according to the trueth, that they haue not any time
before bene touched by the King, to the intent to be healed of that disease. And his Maiestie doth
straitly charge all Iustices of the Peace, Constables and other officers, That they doe not suffer
any to passe, but such as haue such Certificates, vpon paine of his Maiesties displeasure. And to
the end that all his louing Subiects may the better take knowledge of this his Maiesties pleasure
and command, His will is, that this Proclamation be published, and affixed in some open place
in euery Market Towne of this Realme.

Giuen at His Maiesties Court at White-hall, the eighteenth day of Iune, in the second yeere of His Reigne
of Great Britaine, France, and Ireland.

God saue the King.

¶ Imprinted at London by Bonham Norton and Iohn Bill, Printers
to the Kings most Excellent Maiestie. 1626.

FOREWORD

The Royal College of Physicians was founded, by Royal Charter, in 1518 by King Henry VIII. Few professional organisations have been in continuous existence for so long, and over its five-hundred-year history the College has been at the centre of many aspects of medical life. Its purpose is to promote the highest standards of medical practice in order to improve health and health care, and its varied work in the field is held in very high regard. Currently, the College has over thirty thousand members and fellows worldwide. Over the years it has accumulated a distinguished library, extensive archives, museum collections of portraits and other treasures, and has been housed in a number of notable buildings. As part of its quincentennial commemoration, a series of ten books has been commissioned. Each book features fifty items, thereby making a total of five hundred, and the series is intended to be a meditation on, and an exploration of, aspects of the College's work and collections over its five-hundred-year history.

In this third volume in the series of reflections on the RCP's history, celebrated writer and academic Paul Strathern provides a series of entertaining descriptions of a group of practitioners from whom the Royal College of Physicians had always done its best to protect the public. These reflections demonstrate how easy it can be to mislead those looking for treatments and cures, and the importance of the College in its attempts to improve standards of care and practice.

The illustrations were chosen by Julie Beckwith and Peter Basham, and Orla Fee also worked on the production and logistics of the project. On behalf of the RCP, I express my sincere gratitude for their hard work and expertise, which have contributed so much to this volume. I finally would like to thank Sian Rance, the book designer, for making such an attractive volume, and Little Brown our publisher.

Simon Shorvon —

Simon Shorvon, Harveian Librarian, Royal College of Physicians
Series Editor

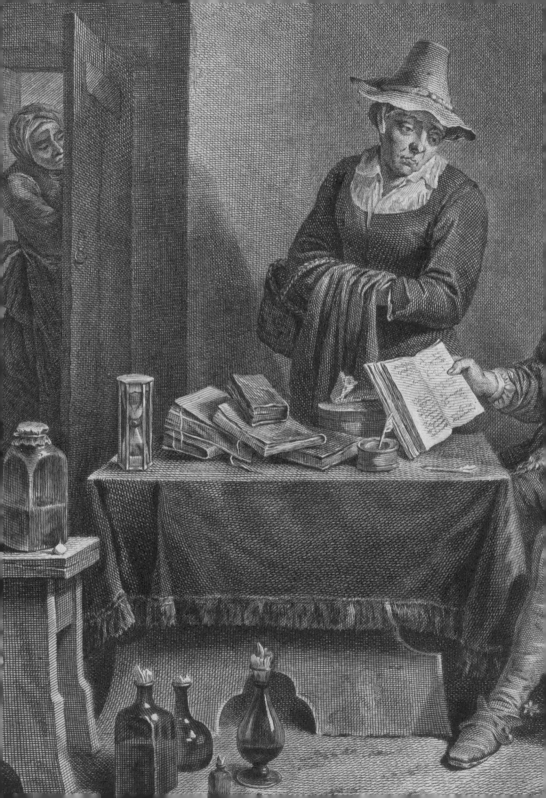

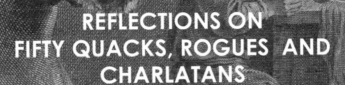

REFLECTIONS ON
FIFTY QUACKS, ROGUES AND
CHARLATANS

The history of the warfare of the physicians against the
quacks is not a story with a plot, a story of strategy,
defeats and victories, leading on to a peace-
settlement; it is an interminable succession of incidents
in which one half of human nature collides
with another.

G. N. Clark *A History of the Royal College of Physicians*

CONTENTS

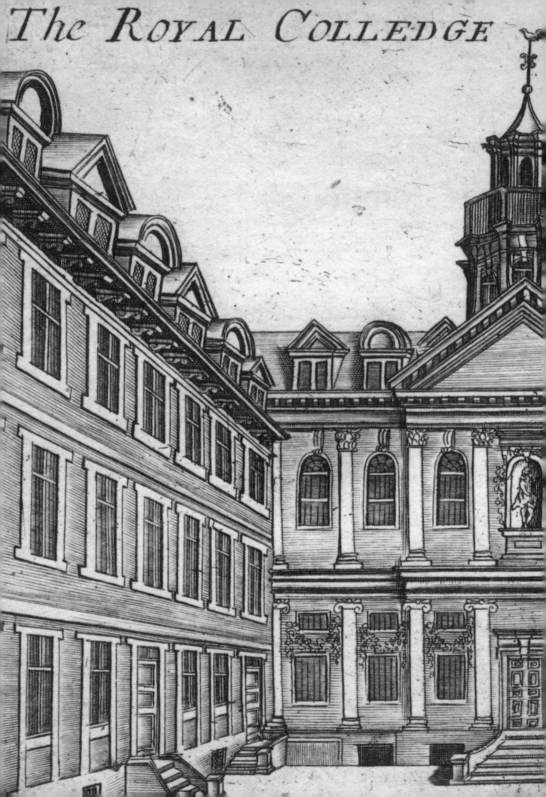

The Royal Colledge

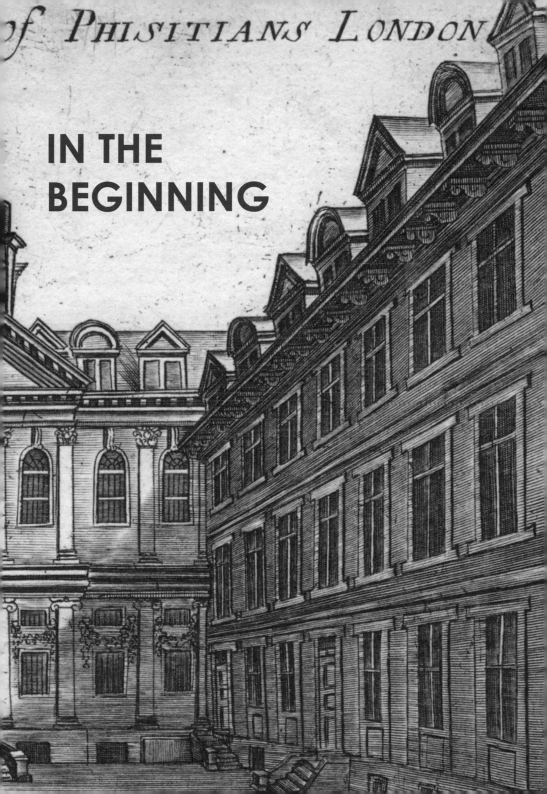

of PHISITIANS LONDON

IN THE
BEGINNING

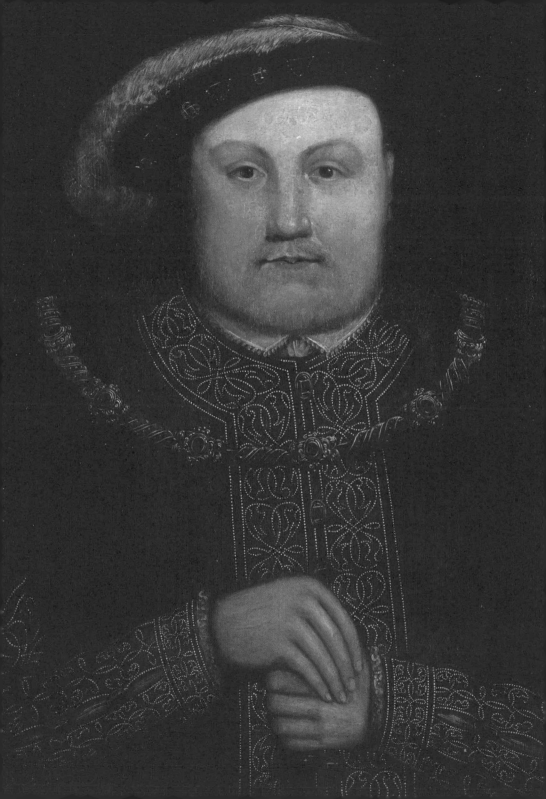

RCP CHARTER

When the Royal College of Physicians was founded during the reign of Henry VIII in 1518, its royal charter specifically indicated the intention:

to curb the audacity of those wicked men who shall profess medicine more for the sake of their avarice than from the assurance of any good conscience, whereby many inconveniences may ensue to the rude and credulous populace.

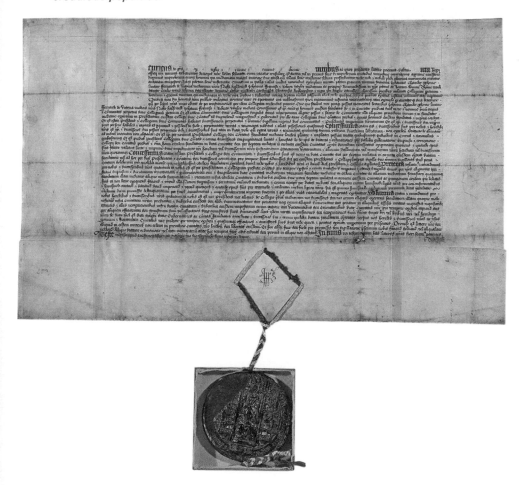

PREVIOUS PAGE: Royal College of Physicians, Warwick Lane
OPPOSITE: Henry VIII
ABOVE: Charter of Incorporation for the College of Physicians under the Great Seal of Henry VIII, 23 September 1518

RCP EXAMINATION OF QUACKS

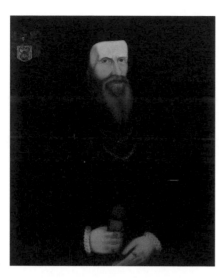

CHAP. XIV.

Of Suppreſſing Quacks.

WHereas there is a great number of unskilful perſons who annoy the Common-wealth, and it lies on us, by the Preſcript of the King and Parliament, that we take care of the health and ſecurity of the people; we appoint and ordain for the more commodious extirpation of ſuch, that whom for certain we ſhall all prove to be unlearned and diſhoneſt,

TOP: John Caius
ABOVE: Extract from the College's byelaws, 1693
OPPOSITE: The case of Alice Leevers, Annals of the College of Physicians, 15 March 1586

Thus, from the very outset a principal aim of the College was the suppression of quacks, frauds and charlatans. In order to eliminate such mountebanks from the ranks of properly licensed practitioners, the Royal College of Physicians would examine those who wished to practise medicine in London, insisting that prior to this they should present evidence of having acquired a medical degree. Such qualifications, even when obtained from the most reputable universities, were not always what they seemed. In 1555 John Caius, who would become master of the Cambridge college which bears his name, complained in a letter to the Vice-Chancellor of Oxford that they had granted an MD (*Medicinae Doctor*) to two men who had been deemed by his college's examiners to be 'illiterate'. In the words of the medical historian Roy Porter: 'In a world where academic honours could legitimately be purchased, possession of a medical degree cannot of itself be taken as proof positive of competence.' Indeed, as we shall see, some charlatans even managed to satisfy the examiners of the Royal College of Physicians, their true status often taking years to come to light (if at all). But such frauds would have been a cut above your common or garden quack, who (despite pretensions) was not regarded as a bona fide member of any profession, other than his own.

From the very outset a principal claim of the College was the suppression of quacks, frauds and charlatans.

In his Comitijs comparuit Alicia Leuers. mulier prorsus im-
perita, et anus delira, longo tamen tempore medicinam ex-
ercens, vt ipsa confitetur. In cuius fauorem literæ
scriptæ ab honoratiss. viro D. Hunsden Regiæ Ma.tis
Domino Cubiculario legebantur: quibus lectis, conclusum
est, vt l̃ræ responsoriæ, rescriberentur, hac quæ
sequitur præscriptione.

l̃ra responso
ria ad Do.
Hunsden

Right honorable and o.r verie good L. whereas it hath pleased
yo.r good L. to send yo.r honorable l̃res in the fauo.r of one Alicia
Leebers, to that effect, that she might be admitted by vs, to
the practise of physick and surgery, Maie it please yo.r Hono.r
to be aduertised, that whereas the said Alicia being a wooman
vtterly ignorant in that profession, for her great erro.rs harmes
and offences that were committed, hath been vtterlie forbidden,
as well by o.r predecessors long time since, as also, diuers othe.r
times of late to by vs, to deale therein: both for that o.r societÿ
is bound by statutes of and continewes, to admonish, correct and
punish all such offendors; and the good lawes likewise of the
Realme, by something hard and streight in that behalf, against
all intruders into a vocation of so great danger, without
sufficient warrant and authority, We therefore most humbly
beseech yo.r good L. to accept of o.r resolution touching the said
party, which is this: That albeit the said Alicia hath contrary
to her owne agreement, and o.r former orders taken herein, medled,
and dailie doth meddle, to the great danger of her Mat.s good
Subiects in that art; wherein she is vtterly ignorant and
therfore hath incurred great punishmente for the same, if extrea-
mitie were vrged: yet seeing it hath pleased yo.r hono.r
to request vs in her behalf, whom in truth yo.r L. may, and
shall, during life, commaund in what so euer, and so doe
beseech yo.r good L. to thinke. we are contented, not onely, fully
to remit all offences heretofore committed by her, touching vs, and

QUACKS IN SOCIETY

The quack, who journeyed the countryside selling all manner of panaceas and 'elixirs' of his own devising, was a common figure in sixteenth-century society. And the resemblance of his name to the noise made by a duck is no coincidence, for in order to advertise his (or her) wares such unlicensed purveyors were forced to go about the streets 'quacking for patients'. The word quack itself is said to derive from the Dutch word *kwakzalver* (loosely 'a common fellow who walks about the place advertising his own concocted medicines by shouting'). Over the coming years such 'quacks' would acquire all manner of detractors. Defoe saw through them at once, describing them as 'ignorant fellows, quacking and tampering in Physick'. Shakespeare's racy friend Ben Jonson, never one to mince words, characterised a quack as 'a turdy-facy, nasty-paty, lousy fartical rogue'.

Prior to the advent of the printing press, quacks relied upon the power and persuasiveness of their voice to advertise their business and attract customers, but come the sixteenth century such self-advertisement was reinforced by the distribution

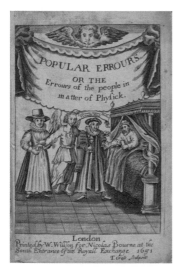

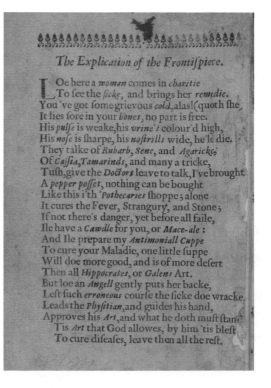

ABOVE: Title page of James Primerose's *Popular Errours*, 1651. It shows a sick man attended by a doctor while an angel stops a quack from intervening
RIGHT: Explanation of the title page of *Popular Errours*
OPPOSITE: A quack doctor selling his treatments (Wellcome Library, London)

218   PUNCH, OR THE LONDON CHARIVARI.   [NOVEMBER 11, 1893,

DR. DULCAMARA UP TO DATE; OR, WANTED A QUACK-QUELCHER.

["The jury, in giving their verdict, strongly censured the gross ignorance of the accused, and regretted that there was no law to prevent them from practising surgery."]

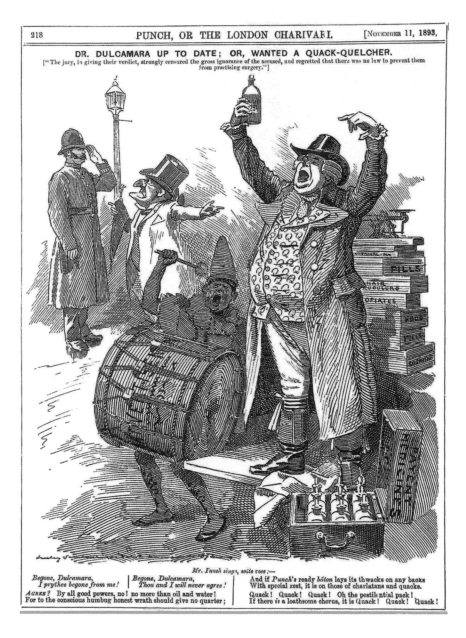

Mr. Punch sings, sotto voce :—

Begone, Dulcamara, | Begone, Dulcamara, | And if *Punch's* ready *bâton* lays its thwacks on any backs
   I prythee begone from me! | Thou and I will never agree! | With special zest, it is on those of charlatans and quacks.
AGREE? By all good powers, no! no more than oil and water! | Quack! Quack! Quack! Oh the pestilential pack!
For to the conscious humbug honest wrath should give no quarter; | If there is a loathsome chorus, it is Quack! Quack! Quack!

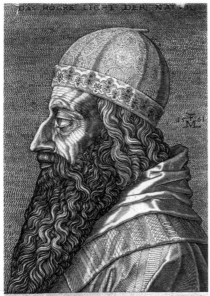

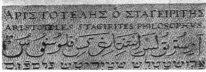

ABOVE: Aristotle
OPPOSITE: Advertisement for a quack doctor, 1650
(© The British Library Board, 1141.a.37.(3))

of cheaply printed and easily circulated hand-bills. An early bill from 1525 promises a cure for: 'The Canker or the Colyck and the Skarre in the lyppe or other diseases in the mouth…Also, if any man hade any dysease in his eyes who be with Spurblindness or a Wem or any other Skynne over the Syghts…' and so on. As Porter confirms, over the coming years: 'Tavern walls were plastered with their bills; people pored over them in coffee houses; their advertisements screamed out from newspapers.'

Yet not all such unlicensed practitioners were outright frauds. The Elizabethan scholar Francis Bacon believed that scientific truth was reached by empirical methods, rather than by scholarly learning, stressing: 'By far the best proof is experience'. Conducting experiments, instead of accepting the authority of classical authors, was the way to arrive at the truth. This was the era which saw the beginnings of the Scientific Revolution. Consequently astronomy began to separate from astrology, chemistry started to break away from alchemy and medical practice gradually cast off the restraints of medieval orthodoxy – which looked to the authority of classical authors such as Galen and Aristotle, many of whose theories were simply erroneous. Galen, for instance, based his ideas of human anatomy on the dissection of monkeys and pigs, as the dissection of human cadavers at the time was forbidden on religious grounds. More than a few of the so-called 'quacks', 'who had never paced the quadrangles of a college', had acquired a wide range of genuine knowledge in the course of their travels.

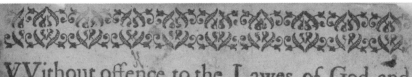

VVithout offence to the Lawes of God and

Man : onely by Mathematicall Arts and Naturall Sciences : A certaine true and probable Anſwer may be given to any lawfull demaund whatſoever, as by the teſtimony of the Learned among all Nations, and in all ages, and innumerable Examples of our owne experience have invincibly confirmed.

1 OF the Complexion of the body : and the Inclination of the minde.
2 Of Riches, and poverty, how, and when they ſhall happen.
3 Of Marriage, the number, quality, time, and place.
4 Of Children, if few, or many, their ſexe and diſpoſition.
5 Of Travailes, the time, the part of the World, and the event.
6 Of the Profeſſion, Trade, and maner of life.
7 Of Dignity, grace, and diſgrace, and from whom.
8 Of Friends and Enemies, and the event of their love or hatred.
9 Whether any that is Abſent be alive ? how ? and where ?
10 Whether any ſhall have riches, and at what time ?
11 Whether a Partner or Factor be juſt and faithfull ?
12 Whether a Man ſhall marry that Woman he deſireth ?
13 Whether a Woman be apt to have Children ?
14 Whether a Man ſhall obtaine what he hopeth for ?
15 Whether a Man ſhall prevaile in his Law-ſuite ?
16 Whether a Man ſhall thrive by the Trade he followeth ?
17 Whether the ſickneſſe be curable or mortall ? alſo I have ready prepared the moſt approved Remedies for all diſeaſes whether outward or inward that are curable.
18 That I have recovered the 3 yeeres dumbe to perfect ſpeech, cured the dead palſie, the falling ſickneſſe, Morbus gallicus, confirmed dangerous Vlcers and Fiſtulaes. Shall bee apparently proved both by oath, and the teſtimonies of Honourable Perſonages.

From my Houſe neere Fetter-lane in Gun-powder Alley, the next doore to Maſter *Corderoy*.

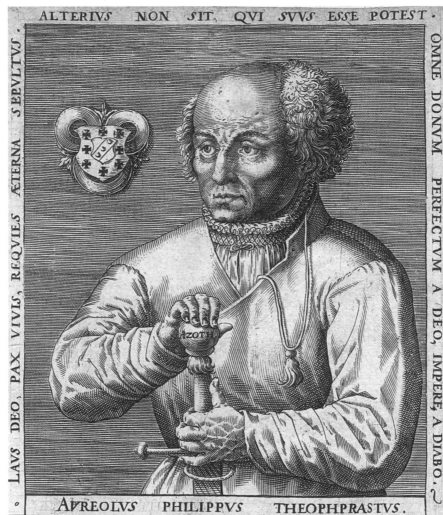

ALTERIVS NON SIT, QVI SVVS ESSE POTEST.

OMINE DONVM PERFECTVM À DEO, IMPERE À DIABO.

LAVS DEO, PAX VIVIS, REQVIES ÆTERNA SEPVLTVS.

AVREOLVS PHILIPPVS THEOPHPRASTVS.

Epitaphium D. Theophraſ.Paracelſi, quod Saliſburgæ in Noſocomio apud S.Sebaſtianum, ad templi murum erectum ſpectatur, lapidi inſculptum

Conditur hic Philippus Theophraſtus inſignis Medicinæ Doctor, qui dira illa Vulnera, Lepram, Podagram, Hidropiſim, alia'que inſanabilia corporis contagia, mirifica arte ſuſtulit, ac bona ſua in pauperes diſtribuenda collocanda'que honorauit. Anno M.D.XXXXI.die xxiiii.Septembris, Vitam cum morte mutauit.

ABOVE: Paracelsus

PARACELSUS

The epitome of this approach can be seen in the sixteenth-century German-Swiss physician Paracelsus, who is regarded throughout much of Continental Europe as 'the father of modern medicine'. An obstreperous character, he was expelled from the University of Ferrara 'for contradicting medical doctrine, ridiculing his teachers, or drunkenness'. Devoid of any academic qualification, he took to the road and became a roving 'student of medicine'. Wherever he went, he would seek out local medicinal lore. Much of this ran contrary to orthodox academic teaching, and he adopted the slogan: 'the more learned, the more perverted'. He ridiculed academic medicine based on the likes of Galen and the renowned ancient Roman physician Celsus. Even the name he took on proclaims his boastful attitude: 'Paracelsus' means 'beyond – or greater than – Celsus'. His real name was Philip Bombastus von Hohenheim, which many believed gave rise to the word 'bombastic', a description that certainly fitted his character.

In Paracelsus' view: 'A doctor must seek out old wives, gypsies, sorcerers, wandering tribes, old robbers and such outlaws and take lessons from them. A doctor must be a traveller…Knowledge is experience.' Medicine was on the cusp. Despite having all the hallmarks of a quack, and not being above the occasional indulgence in the bogus practices associated with this name (especially when he needed some money), Paracelsus was undoubtedly touched with genius. He took medicine seriously and sought to turn it into a genuine science, discarding the outmoded and erroneous practices of the past. And in doing so he accumulated a body of medical knowledge beyond any of his contemporaries. This was the man who may often have slept in a ditch, but he also conversed on equal terms with Erasmus, the leading humanist philosopher of the age, and even cured him of a crippling kidney complaint. Afterwards, Erasmus would say of him: 'I cannot offer thee a fee equal to thine art and learning'. Yet this was also the man who at his inaugural lecture as a professor at the University of Basle (a post obtained for him by Erasmus) chose to dispense with formal academic robes and appeared in a filthy alchemist's leather apron. He announced to his audience of distinguished professors and city authorities that he would reveal to them the greatest secret of medical science. With a flourish, he then removed the cover from the salver on his lectern – to reveal a pile of human excrement.

His students, with whom he enjoyed carousing in the taverns, worshipped his every word. And these were indeed often words of great wisdom. With regard to the excrement he had produced at his inaugural lecture, he claimed: 'If you will not hear the mysteries of putrefactive fermentation, you are unworthy of the name physicians.' Ironically, it was his studies in alchemy which had led him to the pioneering insight that fermentation was a principal feature of our bodily functions. Though not all of his less advertised activities led him to genuine scientific insights. Besides alchemy, Paracelsus is also known to have indulged in astrology and become an avid student of secret hermetic practices. Although he

This curious mixture of the genuinely brilliant and the genuinely bogus would persist well into the coming centuries, in all the sciences.

was undoubtedly a genius, there is no denying that he was also something of a quack, a fraud and a charlatan.

This curious mixture of the genuinely brilliant and the genuinely bogus would persist well into the coming centuries, in all the sciences. Galileo, for instance, practised as an astrologer and was happy to be well rewarded for his troubles. Later still, Newton was a keen adept of alchemy, numerology, biblical divination and all manner of hermetic 'science', utterly convinced that the truth of these pursuits was quite the equal of his mathematical and physical findings. Little wonder, then, that medical practice should continue to attract its fair share of charlatans, of both the self-convinced and the disingenuous variety. (This distinction raises the vexed question of morality where quacks and so forth are concerned. As we shall see, some of the best con-men were those who were utterly convinced of the beneficial effects of their activity; on the other hand, there were always those whose motives were less contaminated by such delusions. In the main, I shall concentrate upon the actions of these figures, rather than attempt any psychological unravelling of tangled motive.)

Paracelsus' travels throughout Europe took him from Scandinavia to Constantinople. According to his biographer, Philip Ball, on many occasions his behaviour led to him being run out of town, 'ascribing his troubles to the jealousy of local physicians, whom he seems to have treated as incompetent cheats'. He certainly visited London, but he seems to have escaped the attentions of the newly formed Royal College of Physicians, who would certainly have curtailed at once the activities of such an unlicensed and bumptious foreign interloper. As we have seen, according to the College's initiating royal charter it was granted the exclusive right to license physicians and, according to Porter, 'unlicensed practitioners could be summoned to answer charges before its court, and even barred from practice and punished'.

This was not quite such a drastic curtailment as it may sound, for initially the Royal College of Physicians only had jurisdiction within the City of London and some seven miles beyond its boundaries – in practice, anywhere within easy walking distance of the largest concentration in the land of moneyed citizens of the 'rude and credulous populace'. Or so it might have seemed. In reality, such was the looseness of this jurisdiction that quacks caught hawking their wares among, say, the vegetable stalls of Cheapside or tailors' shops of Threadneedle Street, would simply repair across London Bridge to Southwark, the unruly district beyond the City boundary which was notorious for its 'stews' (brothels) and unlicensed theatres, like the Globe where Shakespeare's plays found a lively and knowledgeable audience.

SIMON FORMAN

One of the most notorious cases involving such practice was that of Simon Forman, a self-proclaimed 'wizard', who practised the arts of astrology, alchemy and magick – for a suitable fee from his gullible 'patients'. Not content with limiting himself to occult practices, he also found a method of indulging his seemingly insatiable sexual drive. He claimed to have an infallible cure for sexual disorders suffered by women. His method involved taking them to his bed for the night, after which all parties appeared to agree that a cure had taken place. Forman had practised his trade with some vigour for a number of years in the provinces before he ventured into London. It took two years before his methods came to the notice of the Royal College of Physicians, whereupon he was marched off to face their Censors. Here he was charged with falsely claiming to cure 'many Hectical [sic] and tabid people by the use of an Electuary made with rose juice and wormwood water'. The Censors took this matter seriously and he was fined £5, but he refused to pay. He was then sent to prison, but his release was ordered by none other than the Lord Keeper, a senior officer of the Crown, a (male) member of whose family Forman had successfully treated. Whereupon, Forman took the traditional route south across the river, where he 'continued to practise astrology and fortune-telling'. No further mention is made of his 'sexual cure', and he is even said to have got married (possibly for the third time and almost certainly bigamously). In 1611, at the age of fifty-nine, he predicted to his wife that

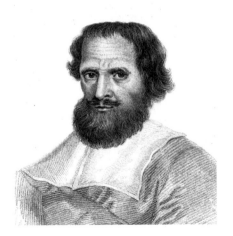

he would die in a drowning accident in the Thames on 12 September. And some months later this duly took place – though as he was dying he is said to have claimed vehemently that the entire accident had been an imposture.

Even so, the Royal College of Physicians was a force to be reckoned with, and took its anti-quackery duties very seriously, strictly adhering to the letter of (its own) law. As a result, it soon began clashing with other similar groups, which often rather more threatened its commercial interests than its enforcement of good practice. In the view of the Royal College of Physicians, the apothecaries (chemists or pharmacists) were a hotbed of quacks and charlatans. They not only prepared their own medicines, thus cutting into the physicians' rich source of income from their own 'preparations', but also gave advice on which medicines were best taken for which ailments and diseases. This was certainly an intrusion into the physicians' protected territory and such charlatanry could not be tolerated.

PHARMACOPOEIA LONDINENSIS

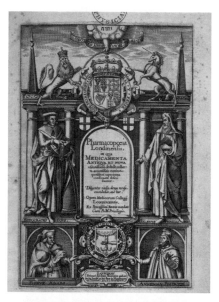

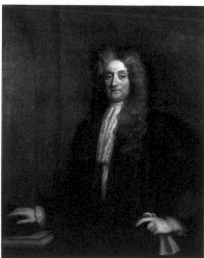

TOP: Title page, *Pharmacopoeia Londinensis*, 2nd ed, 1618
ABOVE: Sir Hans Sloane

The first major clash with the apothecaries as a whole came after the Worshipful Society of Apothecaries was granted a royal charter by James I in 1617. The Royal College of Physicians replied to this affront a year later by issuing a new edition of *Pharmacopoeia Londinensis* (The London Dispensatory) under the presidency of Sir Hans Sloane, the first medical practitioner to receive a hereditary title. The *Pharmacopoeia* was the extensive and definitive volume which specified the precise ingredients and preparations of all licensed medicines, and required the apothecaries, by royal decree, to adhere to these formulas. Unfortunately, such an order was not quite so straightforward as it appeared. The early Latin versions of the *Pharmacopoeia* contained all manner of mistakes, outmoded 'medicines' culled from previous similar works, erroneous instructions and ingredients, as well as wholly false and dangerous claims. Some medicines were even listed as being able 'to cure poison'. Such claims may have been acceptable in an earlier time, but medicine was now moving into the modern scientific age, consequently many entries themselves now bordered on sheer quackery, to say the least. Ingredients included 'dog's excrement', 'earth worms' and 'moss from the human skull'. Consequent editions, which attempted to correct these errors, as well as various pirated 'translations' into English, along with unauthorised 'commentaries' inserted by their various translators, only served to muddy the waters still further. As the College

Many entries themselves now bordered on sheer quackery, to say the least. Ingredients included 'dog's excrement', 'earth worms' and 'moss from the human skull'.

itself would later admit, it was not until 'the 1745 and 1788 revisions of the *Pharmacopocia* [that] some semblance of rationality began to appear'.

Yet miraculously, this sorry tale would have a happy outcome. Despite the endless wranglings, the publication of *Pharmacopoeia Londinensis* (and its consequent amended editions) was to prove a landmark in medicine. For the first time, medicines were licensed and named, their ingredients and preparation precisely specified. All other medicines were de facto the elixirs of quacks, or even poisons. This work would prove a forerunner for the College's 'Nomenclature of Diseases', first published in 1869, and subsequently accepted worldwide. Doing for medicine what Linnaeus had done for the world's flora and fauna, this work would only be superseded in the twentieth century by the World Health Organisation's *Manual of international classification of diseases*.

Over the years the Royal College of Physicians would find itself involved in similar long-standing clashes with surgeons, obstetricians and others, all medical practices which attracted their measure of quacks, frauds and charlatans. Such disputes might not always have been conducted in the most effective fashion, or with the purest of motives, but they served a purpose in the elimination of fake medical practices.

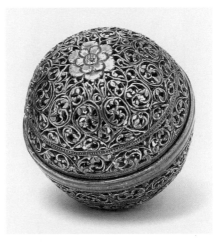

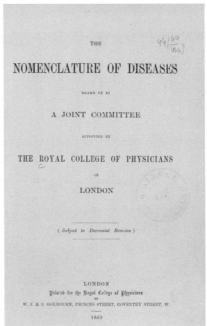

THE

NOMENCLATURE OF DISEASES

DRAWN UP BY

A JOINT COMMITTEE

APPOINTED BY

THE ROYAL COLLEGE OF PHYSICIANS

OF

LONDON

(*Subject to Decennial Revision*)

LONDON
Printed for the Royal College of Physicians
BY
W. J. & S. GOLBOURN, PRINCES STREET, COVENTRY STREET, W.
1869

TOP: Silver bezoar stone box, late 17th century. Bezoar stones were used as antidotes to poison
ABOVE: Title page of the Royal College of Physicians' *The Nomenclature of Diseases*, 1869

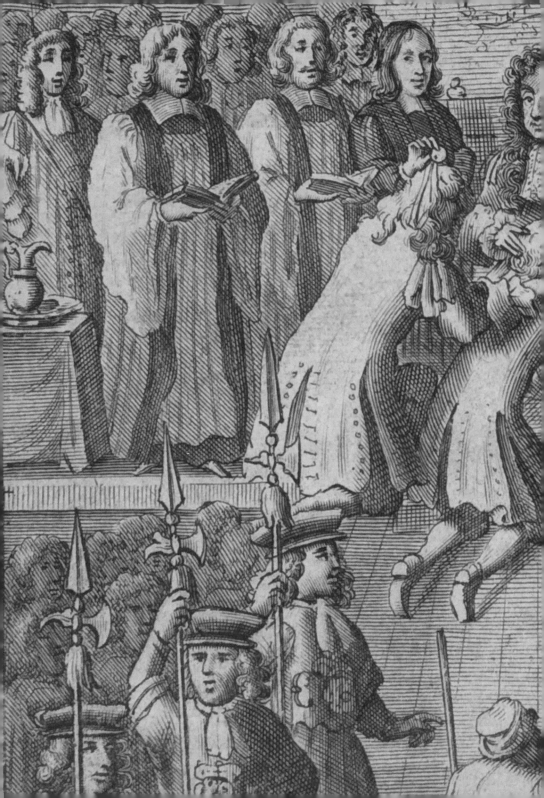

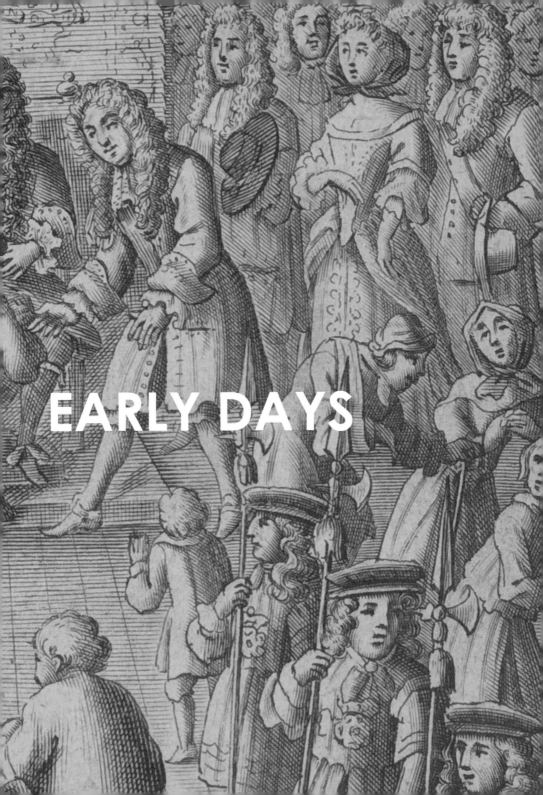

EARLY DAYS

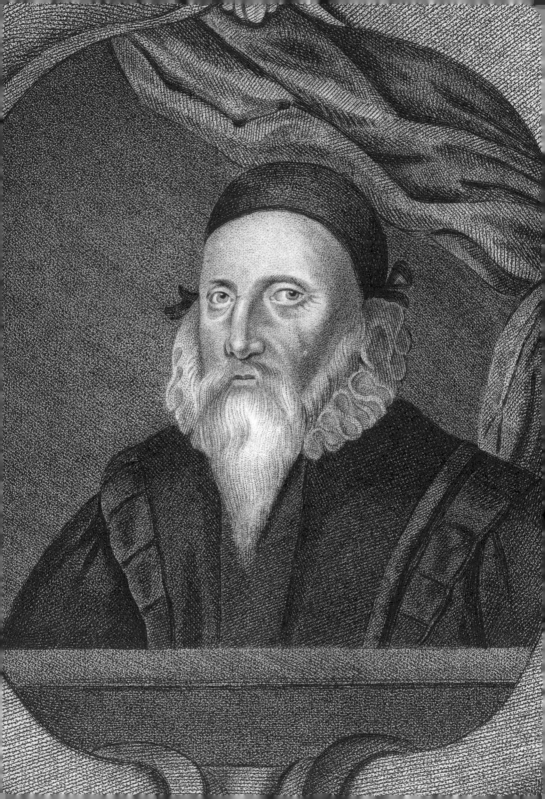

With the founding of the Royal College of Physicians in 1518, all those who practised medicine without a licence from the College automatically fell into the category of quacks or charlatans, with their elixirs and potions being adjudged frauds. However, the College would find it expedient to turn a blind eye with regard to some who belonged in this category.

JOHN DEE

Take, for example, that quintessential Elizabethan genius John Dee, who was a physician to Queen Elizabeth I, as well as being her trusted advisor (his astrological expertise was used to choose her coronation day). Much like his accomplished contemporary Paracelsus, Dee's scholarly pursuits were far too wide-ranging to remain confined within the bounds of purely orthodox enquiry. Dee was a man of his age, when astrology and astronomy, mathematics and divination, to say nothing of both Aristotelian and hermetic philosophy, all remained objects of intellectual enquiry. Regardless of his high post as a physician, Dee was never in fact invited to join the Royal College of Physicians. And in hindsight, this would prove an astute omission, when Dee was 'subsequently derided as a conjuror and a trickster'.

Despite this, today the College library is proud to contain the largest collection of books from Dee's famous library including alchemical texts annotated in his own hand and a work by the legendary mage Hermes Trismegistus. (Regardless of the subject matter of some of the volumes in Dee's collection: even the collection itself is not without its controversial aspect, as 'several of the volumes contain evidence which shows that a subsequent owner, Sir Nicholas Saunder, was a thief or a receiver of books stolen during Dee's absence abroad in the 1580s'.)

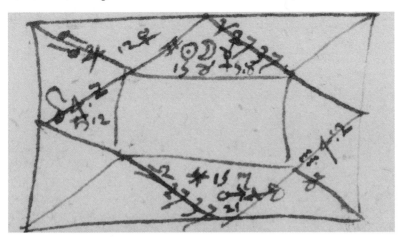

PREVIOUS PAGE: Charles II touch ceremony. In John Browne's *Adenochoiradelogia*, 1684
ABOVE: A horoscope annotation by John Dee. In Ptolemy (and others) *Quadriparti...*, 1519
OPPOSITE: John Dee

THE ROYAL TOUCH

Strictly speaking Elizabeth I herself was also a quack, in that she indulged in the practice known as the Royal Touch. This is precisely what it sounds like, and was said to cure any subject, from a royal prince to the lowliest commoner, of the disease known as scrofula (tuberculosis). The practice was said to date back to Henry III, who reigned in the thirteenth century. The Royal Touch took on a particular significance whenever the monarch felt under threat, as this miraculous ability was said to demonstrate the monarch's divine right – in other words, the fact that he received his authority from God and ruled according to His will. This ritual assumed supreme importance during the rule of Charles II, whose father had been deposed and beheaded, despite insisting on his divine right to rule. So keen was Charles II to demonstrate

The Royal Touch took on a particular significance whenever the monarch felt under threat.

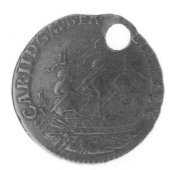

his powers that during the course of his twenty-five-year reign he is said to have 'touched' more than 92,000 of his subjects (which accounted for almost one in fifty of the population).

The divinity of the Royal Touch was said to be confirmed by the Bible, where the Gospel according to St Mark claims that monarchs are immune from infectious diseases and that 'they shall lay hands on the sick and they shall recover'. James I, who succeeded Elizabeth I (but did not retain the services of John Dee), appears to have placed less faith in St Mark's claim and fastidiously refused to touch any of his scrofulous citizens, choosing instead merely to wave his hand over their heads. When the rather more down-to-earth Dutch king William III ascended to the throne of Britain in 1689, he dismissed the practice as simply superstition, refusing a petitioner with the words: 'God grant you better health and better sense'. However, his successor Queen Anne enthusiastically revived the practice, to such an extent that on 30 March 1712 she 'touched' 300 people, including the infant Samuel Johnson.[1] However, the records show that quite a number of those who were 'touched' did experience a degree of cure. This may have been due to psychosomatic causes induced by awe of the royal presence, or the fact that scrofula often went into spontaneous remission. The Royal Touch was not abandoned until the succession in 1714 of the Hanoverian George I, who applied some German common

ABOVE: Charles II touchpiece. Touchpieces were given by the monarch to those they touched. They were pierced so that they could be worn on a ribbon around the neck
OPPOSITE: Royal touch: a proclamation, 1683

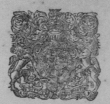

109/49.

At the Court at WHITEHALL

The Ninth of *January* 1 6 8 3.

Prefent

The Kings moſt Excellent Majeſty,

Lord Keeper	*Earl of* Huntingdon	*Earl of* Bathe	*Mr. Secretary* Jenkins
Lord Privy Seal	*Earl of* Bridgewater	*Earl of* Craven	*Mr. Chancellour of the* Exchequer
Duke of Ormond	*Earl of* Peterborrow	*Earl of* Nottingham	*Mr. Chancellour of the* Dutchy
Duke of Beaufort	*Earl of* Cheſterfield	*Earl of* Rocheſter	*Lord Chief Juſtice* Jeffryes
Earl of Oxford	*Earl of* Clarendon	*Lord Biſhop of* London	*Mr.* Godolphin.

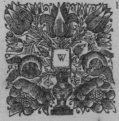

Hereas by the Grace and Bleſſing of God, the Kings and Queens of this Realm by many Ages paſt, have had the happineſs by their Sacred Touch, and Invocation of the Name of God, to cure thoſe who are afflicted with the Diſeaſe called the Kings-Evil; And His Majeſty in no leſs meaſure than any of His Royal Predeceſſors having had good ſucceſs therein, and in His moſt Gracious and Pious diſpoſition, being as ready and willing as any King or Queen of this Realm ever was in any thing to relieve the diſtreſſes and neceſſities of His good Subjects; Yet in His Princely Wiſdom foreſeeing that in this (as in all other things) Order is to be obſerved, and fit times are neceſſary to be appointed for the performing of this great work of Charity, His Majeſty was therefore this day pleaſed to Declare in Council His Royal Will and Pleaſure to be, That (in regard heretofore the uſual times of preſenting ſuch perſons for this purpoſe have been prefixed by His Royal Predeceſſors) the times of Publick Healings ſhall from henceforth be from the Feaſt of *All Saints*, commonly called *Alhallon-tide*, till a week before *Chriſtmas* : and after *Chriſtmas* until the Firſt day of *March*, and then to ceaſe till the *Paſſion Week*, being times moſt convenient both for the temperature of the ſeaſon, and in reſpect of Contagion which may happen in this near acceſs to His Majeſties Sacred Perſon. And when His Majeſty ſhall at any time think fit to go any Progreſs, He will be pleaſed to appoint ſuch other times for Healing as ſhall be moſt convenient : And His Majeſty doth hereby accordingly Order and Command, That from the time of Publiſhing this His Majeſties Order, none preſume to repair to His Majeſties Court to be Healed of the ſaid Diſeaſe, but onely at, or within the times for that purpoſe hereby appointed as aforeſaid. And His Majeſty was further pleaſed to Order, That all ſuch as hereafter ſhall come, or repair to the Court for this purpoſe, ſhall bring with them Certificates under the Hands and Seals of the Parſon, Vicar, or Miniſter, and of both or one of the Churchwardens of the reſpective Pariſhes where they dwell, and from whence they come, teſtifying according to the truth, That they have not at any time before been touched by His Majeſty to the intent to be healed of that Diſeaſe. And all Miniſters and Churchwardens are hereby required to be very careful to examine into the truth before they give ſuch Certificates, and alſo to keep a Regiſter of all Certificates they ſhall from time to time give. And to the end that all His Majeſties Loving Subjects may the better take knowledge of this His Majeſties Command, His Majeſty was pleaſed to Direct, That this His Order be Read publickly in all Pariſh-Churches, and then be affixt to ſome conſpicuous place there; And that to that end the ſame be Printed, and a convenient Number of Copies ſent to the moſt Reverend Fathers in God, the Lord Arch Biſhop of *Canterbury*, and the Lord Arch Biſhop of *York*, who are to take care that the ſame be diſtributed to all Pariſhes within their reſpective Provinces.

PHI. LLOYD.

LONDON,

Printed by the Aſſigns of *John Bill* Deceas'd : And by *Henry Hills*, and *Thomas Newcomb*, Printers to the Kings moſt Excellent Majeſty. 1683.

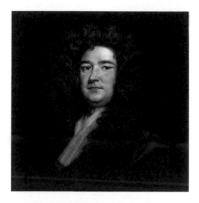

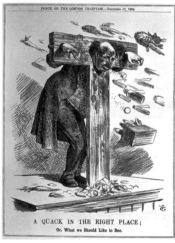

A QUACK IN THE RIGHT PLACE;
Or, What we Should Like to See.

TOP: Sir Richard Blackmore
ABOVE: A quack in the right place; or what we should like to see (Wellcome Library, London)

The Royal Touch had long been regarded with some scepticism by the Royal College of Physicians, but owing to their establishment by royal charter this placed them in an invidious position

sense to the matter and banished the practice. The noted contemporary physician Sir Richard Blackmore praised this move for putting an end to a 'superstitious ceremony' which he ascribed to a 'Popish plot'. Understandably, the Royal Touch had long been regarded with some scepticism by the Royal College of Physicians, but owing to their establishment by royal charter this placed them in an invidious position, consequently no public pronouncement was made on this topic.

Straightforward quackery, plain and simple, has usually been found in minor practitioners – from early panacea-sellers to snake oil salesmen and modern 'healers'.[2] Those 'mountebanks too piffling' to warrant the attention of the Royal College of Physicians were liable to be apprehended by the local magistrates and placed in the stocks. This was a painful and humiliating experience which often involved much more than the boisterous pelting with rotten vegetables, so beloved of popular folklore. Amid crowd hysteria, the victim could often become a scapegoat for deeper social grievances. Hurled faeces could infect open wounds; disguised stones could crack skulls or even knock out an eye; and any sentence of longer than one day could involve near starvation or severe illness from exposure to the elements.

CHARLES CORNET

In 1555, one quack who was lucky to escape this fate was Charles Cornet, who according to a contemporary report was:

> *an impudent and ignorant Buffoon, who would not be restrained from his ill practises [sic], with the bills of his condemnation affixed at the corners of streets…was forced to flee the town and had his unwholesome remedies burnt in the open market at Westminster.*

TOMAZINE SCARLET, STIBIUM AND SNAKE OIL

And female quacks were not unknown. In 1588, Tomazine Scarlet:

> *a woman so egregiously ignorant that she confessed she knew nothing of Physick, neither could reade or write, yet had hundreds under her cure to whom she gave medicines, Stibium, etc., was charged with base practices. She was fined Ten pounds and was committed to prison for her mis-deeds.*

This contemporary report might not be all that it seems. Ten pounds was double the annual wage of a craftsman – a heavy fine, probably reflecting Scarlet's popularity among so many clients. And some have suggested that the fact she used stibium, a concoction of antimony popular with alchemists, indicates she may well have been practising 'Paracelsian medicine'. In which case, her illiteracy and ignorance of 'Physick' would certainly have been feigned. All of this indicates that the Royal College of Physicians had a hand in this prosecution.

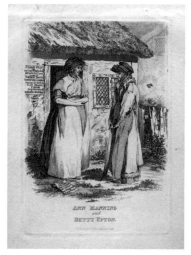

Ann Manning, a quack doctress shown outside her cottage with Betty Upton

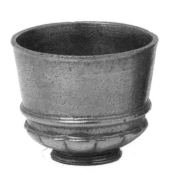

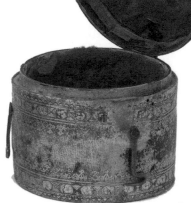

Antimony cup, 1630s

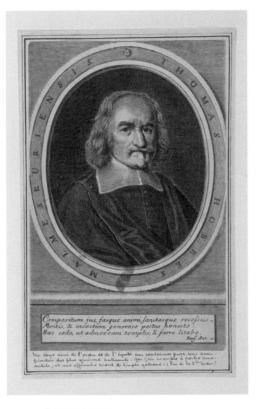

Compossitum jus fasque animi sanctosque recessius
Mentis, & incoctum generoso pectus honesto
Hac cedo, ut admoveam templis, & farre litabo.

Thomas Hobbes

THOMAS HOBBES AND ROBERT . SOUTHEY

Such quackery tended to find favour among the common populace, who were not only more gullible but could also not afford the services of a physician licensed by the College. However, licensed physicians were not universally popular, even among men of the highest learning. This can be seen from the claim by the philosopher Thomas Hobbes: 'I would rather have the advice, or take physick from an experienced old woman that had been at many sick people's bedsides than from the learnedst but inexperienced physician.' Even a century later, the poet laureate Robert Southey noted that 'a cunning man, or a cunning woman, as they are termed, is to be found near every town'. Hobbes was far from being alone among intellectuals attracted to such figures.

'I would rather have the advice, or take physick from an experienced old woman that had been at many sick people's bedsides than from the learnedst but inexperienced physician.'

AN UNFORTUNATE CASE

However, there were occasions when the Censors of the Royal College of Physicians only muddied the waters still further in such matters. Most notable in this aspect is the case of Dr Thomas Bonham, who had studied medicine at both Oxford and Cambridge before travelling south around 1610 with the intention of setting up practice in London. He applied to the Royal College for a licence, 'but was rejected and told to return after further study'. When Bonham chose to disregard this judgement, he was hauled before the College Censors and flung into Newgate Jail for contempt. There followed a lengthy and tedious series of trials, appeals, and counter-trials, before various courts, during the course of which verdicts were reached both for and against Bonham, who became a sort of whipping boy for lawyers, judges, parliamentarians and the King, all of whom claimed that the case lay within their jurisdiction. Bonham's trial would make legal history, causing judges to make a number of learned legal pronouncements concerning precedents, some of whose precise interpretation has yet to be decided to this day.

JAMES THEMUT AND FALLING SICKNESS

In 1660, a man calling himself 'James Themut a native of Vienna in Austria' appeared in the university city of Oxford, where he took up residence at the Saracen tavern. From here he began distributing hand-bills advertising himself as a physician who could cure all manner of illnesses, such as 'falling sickness, Madness, Phrensie and Giddiness in the head…Stinking breath, rotten teeth, Scurvey or Water canker.' As well as this, he had a particular ability to remedy 'secret diseases of Women and Maids' and even 'Morbidus Gallicus' (the French disease, or syphilis). According to a contemporary: 'The vulgar are apt to admire strangers & they also flocked to this man & left the University physitians'. However, 'a month after this man's coming, he ran away & coseneth his patients of a great quantity of money yt [that] he had taken of them before hand'. Among the many undergraduates and scholars he conned was the young Earl of Rochester, who would go on to become an accomplished, if decidedly racy, poet whose work much amused his friend Charles II.

ALEXANDER BENDO, 'NOBLE MOUNTEBANK'

The experience of being conned led Rochester to publish seven years later a pamphlet entitled 'The Famous Pathologist of the Noble Mountebank'. This outlined the antics of the 'Imortal Dr Alexand^r Bendo', who after various scrapes in Italy and France ended up taking on his present name and establishing himself at Tower Street in London. It told how he offered 'for Certain Cure of all sorts of distempers, Malladies and Complaints whatsoever', describing 'his free and open way of making his Medicines in the View of all sorts of People, that pleas'd to come to his Laboratory, he hourly received good Gold and Silver, which was Chearfully paid him, by his credulous Patients wth thanks to boot; for his Affable and communicative Advise.'

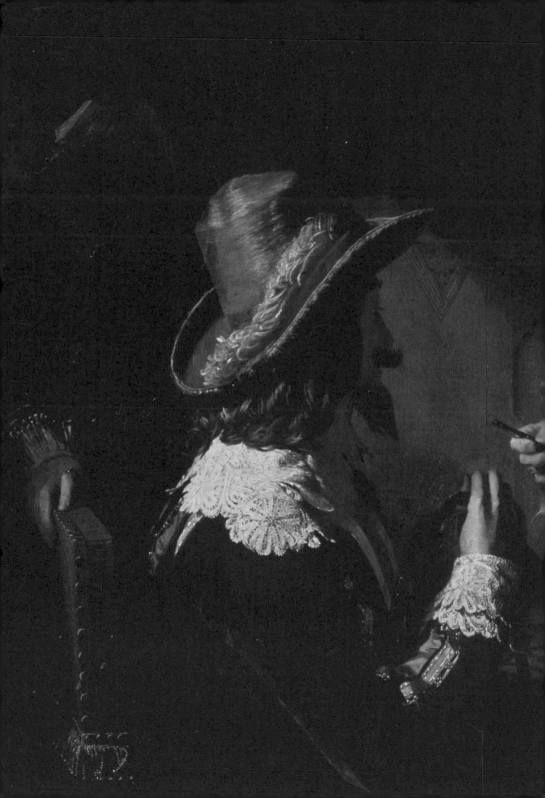

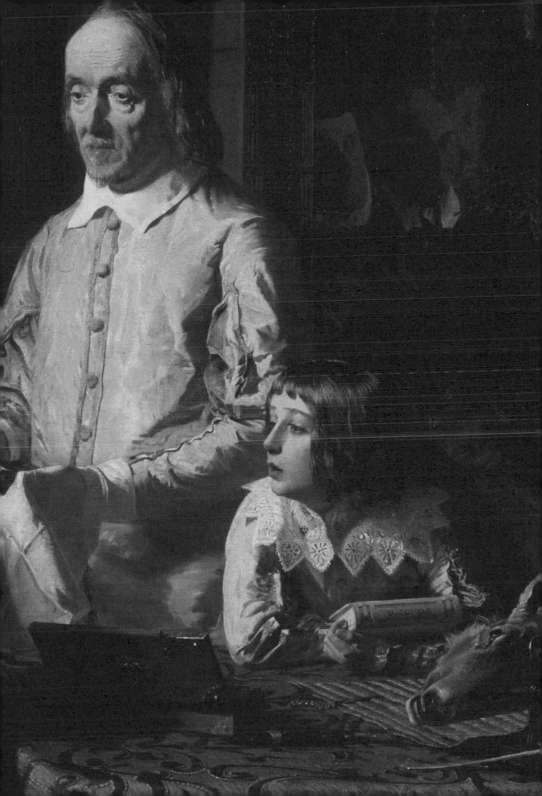

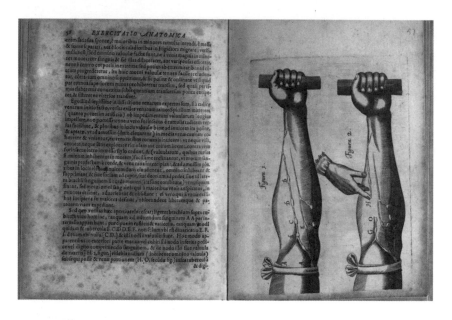

WILLIAM HARVEY, 'THE CIRCULATOR'

One of the early, and most distinguished, members of the College of Physicians was William Harvey, whose discovery of the circulation of the blood would revolutionise our understanding of the human body. In 1615, Harvey had become a lecturer at the Royal College of Physicians, some years after returning from Padua, where he had studied under the celebrated Italian anatomist Hieronymus Fabricius. Harvey was a quick-tempered personality who was liable to whip out a dagger from the sheath on his belt if any dared to cross him. However, when it came to his medicine he was hardly as forthcoming as his dagger. And as we shall see, he had good reason for this. One cannot in all seriousness claim that the great William Harvey was a fraud, yet for many years his behaviour was undeniably duplicitous, to say the least. His revolutionary ideas concerning the circulation of the blood by the pumping of the heart were already fully formed by the time he came to lecture at the Royal College of Physicians. Yet throughout the ensuing years he would continue to teach his students the orthodox, but erroneous Galenic explanation of how the body worked. According to this, the blood was continuously created by the liver, whereupon it flowed through the body and was consumed by the flesh – a one-way system.

Not until 1628 did Harvey venture to publish his seminal work *De Motu Cordis* (Concerning the Motion of the Heart) and even then he chose to have it printed abroad

PREVIOUS PAGE: William Harvey demonstrating circulation of the blood to Charles I
TOP: William Harvey's *De motu cordis*, 1628

in Frankfurt. When copies finally began reaching England, his early biographer Aubrey described how 'twas beleeved by the vulgar that he was crack-brained; and all the Physitians were against his Opinion'. Word got about that Harvey was no more than a quack. His lucrative private practice suffered badly, and the conservative element in the Royal College of Physicians began referring to him as 'Harvey the circulator' – a double-edged epithet (*circulator* is Latin for quack).

HARVEY'S WITCH

Ironically, the most enthusiastic champion of Harvey's ideas was none other than Hobbes, who certainly knew what he was talking about. Despite his penchant for old wives' cures, Hobbes had attended lectures on medicine in Oxford and Paris, and when he later befriended Harvey, who was the King's physician at the time, they would together carry out autopsies on the King's deer. Harvey was obsessed with dissection and even dissected his wife's dead parrot, discovering inside it an egg, which surprised him since, 'I always thought him to be a Cock-parrat'. And it was this obsession which would lead to him exposing a quack, who has become known as Harvey's witch.

During the course of his duties as the royal physician, Harvey accompanied the King to Newmarket, where according to a contemporary chronicler he was despatched to visit...

a woman who was reputed a witch...who dwelt in a lone House on the borders of the Heath...Hee [i.e. Harvey] said she was very distrustful at first; but when hee told her that he was a vizard, and come purposely to converse with her in their common trade, then shee easily believed him [because of his] very magicall face.

In the course of their conversation, Harvey asked the witch if he could see her 'familiar' – a witch's assistant devil, who took on the form of an animal, such as a black cat. The woman opened a cupboard and called out a toad, for which she set out a saucer of milk. Harvey asked the woman if she could fetch him a pot of ale from the tavern down the road, and the moment she was gone he pounced on the toad and began to dissect it. 'Hee examined the toades entrayles, heart and lungs [which were] no wayes different from other toades...ergo it was a plain naturall toad... From whence he concludes there are no witches very logistically.' As it happened, the woman returned while Harvey was still avidly inspecting the toad's entrails. She at once 'flew like a Tigris at his face [so that] he was in danger to have a more magical face than hee had before'. Harvey was lucky to escape with only a badly scratched face, yet, in the true traditions of the College, he had succeeded in unmasking yet another fraud.

During the period when Harvey held the post of King's physician he was instructed by Charles I to undertake a 'diagnosis of witchcraft', which involved him examining

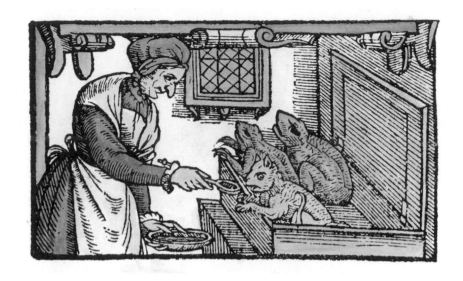

Another for a sore brest or any
swellinge, whitloe, fellon, or byle.
Take new milke from ye cow & small
oatemeales and boyle them together very
well & put in a peece of sweet butter when
it's boyl'd, & soe apply it to ye swellinge &c.

Another for piles
Take white bread & milke & red rose leaues & boyle
them together, then put a litle fat of a calues chaudron
& soe apply it as hot as may be suft red

A good receipt agst witchcraft
Take vermine night shade Dill of each 9 tops,
let all these be strayned together & let ye party
drinke ye juice in white wine, if they feare
the company of any such let them peare it
in their shoes, or under their arms. A poultice for

TOP: A witch feeding familiars
ABOVE: A recipe for witchcraft (MS499)

a number of witches. He remained sceptical with regard to witches' powers, but took the humane view that when a woman was tried for witchcraft it was necessary to prove that she had supernatural powers before she could be convicted (whereupon she would usually be burnt at the stake). In 1634, four women of Lancashire, who had been accused of witchcraft, were brought to London and Harvey presided over an examination of these defendants at their trial. One of the women had confessed to the Bishop of Chester that she had for many years practised witchcraft, while another was found to have two extra teats, apparent evidence that she had 'suckled the devil'. The women were eventually all acquitted, almost certainly on Harvey's instructions. The women had probably been guilty of practising nothing more than old wives' cures.

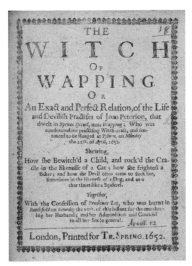

ABOVE: *The Witch of Wapping: the life and devilish practises of Joan Peterson*, 1652. (© The British Library Board, E.659.(18.))

JOAN PETERSON

Alas, a more typical case was that of Joan Peterson. According to a contemporary chronicler:

Joan Peterson, that dwelt in Spruce Island, near Wapping; who was condemned for practising Witch-craft, and sentenced to be hanged at Tyburn, on Munday the 11th. of April, 1652. Shewing, how she bewitch'd a Child, and rock'd the cradle in the likenesse of a Cat; how she frighted a Baker; and how the Devil often came to suck her, sometimes in the likeness of a Dog, and other times like a Squirrel.

Joan had in fact been a popular figure among the residents of Wapping, who came to her for cures of the ague (malaria) and other locally prevalent maladies. When a man refused to pay her for her services, she is said to have put the 'evil eye' on him, whereupon he had a fit. In the absence of any scientific examiner such as Harvey, this evidence was enough to have her condemned.

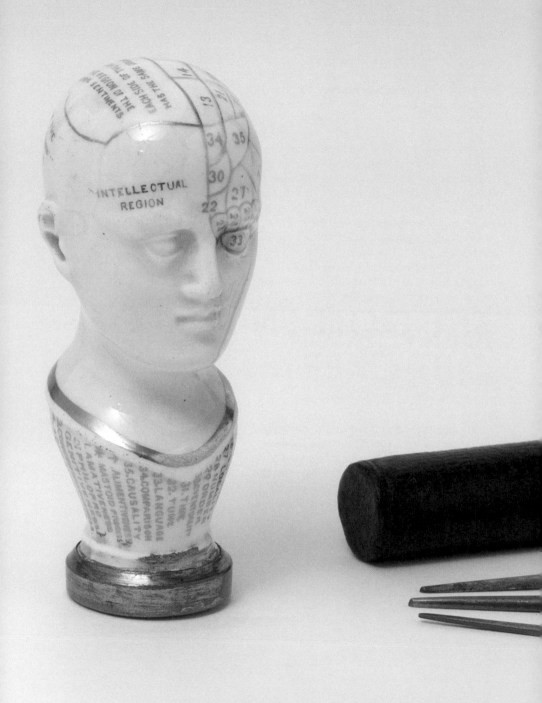

THE GOLDEN AGE OF QUACKERY

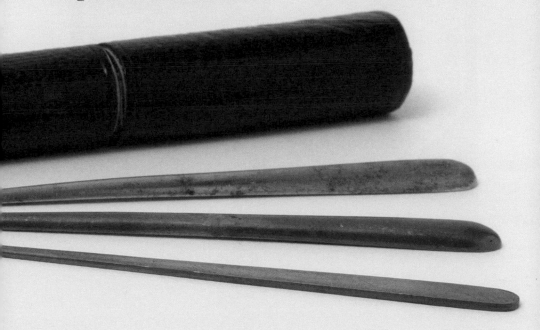

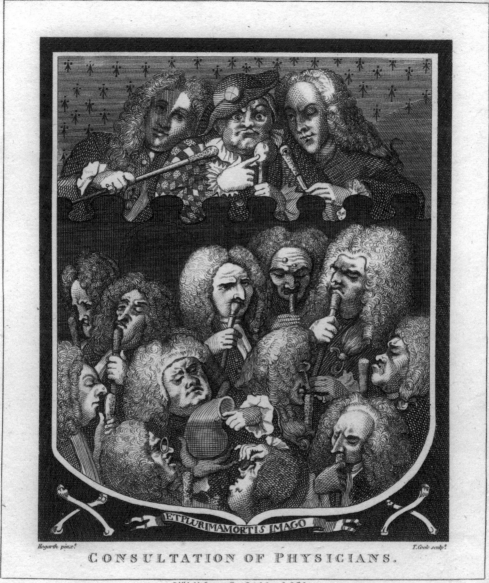

CONSULTATION OF PHYSICIANS.

PREVIOUS PAGE: Phrenology head sea; and galvanic tractors and case
ABOVE: Hogarth's *Consultation of Physicians* ('The Company of Undertakers'). Shown top, left to right, are Chevalier Taylor, Mrs Mapp and Joshua (Spot) Ward
RIGHT: Hogarth's *Marriage à la Mode*: the quack doctor's studio

HOGARTH AND HIS IMAGES OF QUACKS

The early years of the eighteenth century would see the beginning of the Golden Age of Quackery. This was the time of Hogarth, and several of his cartoons would depict quacks – most notably a group portrait satirically entitled 'The Company of Undertakers'. This depicts twelve stout bewigged physicians examining a flask of urine. These are presided over by three immediately identifiable contemporary quacks – Mrs Mapp 'the bonesetter', 'Dr' Joshua 'Spot' Ward and the notorious 'Chevalier' John Taylor. Beneath the group portrait is the Latin motto 'Et plurima mortis imago' (And many an image of death).

This was the time of Hogarth, and several of his cartoons would depict quacks.

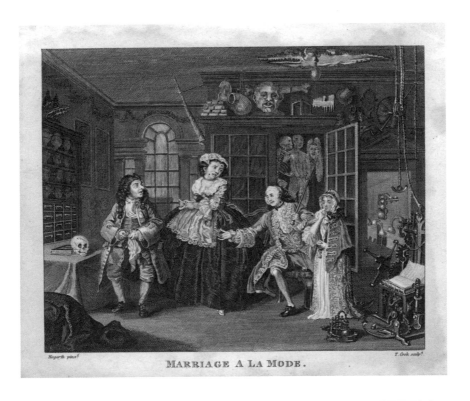

Hogarth pinx.t   T. Cook sculp.t

MARRIAGE A LA MODE.

MRS MAPP

Mrs Mapp, commonly known as 'Crazy Sally', remains something of a divisive figure when it comes to quackery. There is no doubting her considerable abilities as a bonesetter – an art whose secret was passed on to her by her father. This 'secret' consisted in part of manipulative skill, and in part of 'the knack'. The latter she certainly gained through experience. Born and raised in rural Wiltshire during the last years of the seventeenth century, she moved to the market town of Epsom, which was then some fourteen miles outside London. Here she set up manipulating joints, resetting dislocations and aligning bone fractures. Such was her success that people began travelling from London to be treated by 'Crazy Sally', whose 'knack' frequently involved considerable physical strength. It was said that she could reset a shoulder bone single-handed, without even an assistant to hold down her patient.

Afraid of losing their local attraction, the people of Epsom offered her an annual stipend of more than £100 to remain in the town. Although she remained in Epsom, she would take the coach to London twice a week and set up practice at the Grecian Coffee House, off Fleet Street. This was frequented by scientists of the Royal Society, such as Edmund Halley and Sir Hans Sloane, whose niece she successfully treated for a badly broken back.

So why was Mrs Mapp regarded as a quack? To a certain extent this was because the 'art' she practised was unlicensed and held in some contempt by qualified physicians. However, the main reason for her notoriety seems to have stemmed from her looks and her behaviour. 'Crazy Sally' was a woman of formidable ugliness: her big boorish cross-eyed face sat atop the bulky shoulders of a prize-fighter, while her arms were those of a wrestler. She was also something of a tippler and 'is said to have been rarely sober'. If nothing else, she certainly played the role of a brazen quack.

Having made her fortune, 'Crazy Sally' took to travelling up to London in her own horsedrawn coach. On one occasion, while travelling into London up the Old Kent Road, she was mistaken for one of the King's unpopular German mistresses.[3] Her coach was mobbed, until she stuck her head out of the window and yelled: 'Damn your bloods! Don't you know me? I'm Mrs Mapp the bonesetter.' The mob immediately began cheering her on her way.

In 1736 she decided to get married and her fancy alighted on a footman from Ludgate Hill. After their marriage he abused her, and then ran off – supposedly in fear of his life – but taking with him all her money. Her drunkenness eventually got the better of her and she died in poverty in the notorious Seven Dials district of London. A contemporary versifier provided a fitting tribute:

> *Let those, O Mapp, thou wonder of the age!*
> *With dubious arts endeavour to engage;*
> *While you, irregularly strict to rules,*
> *Teach dull collegiate pedants they are fools.*

Although she appears to have been no charlatan or fraud, her demeanour and calling have ensured that no description of the golden age of quackery is complete without Mrs Mapp the bonesetter.

JOSHUA WARD AND RICHARD MEAD

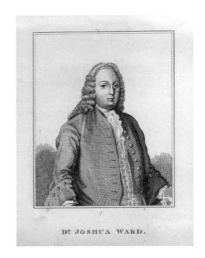

Dʳ JOSHUA WARD.

Her male companions in Hogarth's cartoon, on the other hand, well deserve their place in the rogues' gallery. Dr Joshua 'Spot' Ward was, needless to say, no doctor. (He acquired his nickname from a prominent birthmark on his face). His background is suitably obscure, but he first emerges into the light of day as a pickle-seller on the banks of the Thames. At some stage he disappeared to France, returning in a hurry to avoid imprisonment in the Bastille. Ward was a supreme confidence man and embarked upon his career as such by presenting himself at the Houses of Parliament as the MP for Marlborough. He seems to have fitted in well with his fellow members, for it was several months before he was unmasked. From politics, he turned to medicine. Somehow, probably through purchase from an impecunious medical student, he came into the possession of recipes for the two medicines which would make him famous. These he called 'Ward's Pill and Drop'. The 'pill' was an antimony compound which calmed down feverish patients by all but poisoning them. The 'drop' was a tincture which cured its patients by violently voiding their digestive tract of any contents which might, or might not, have been causing their complaint.

Once Ward discovered that these products 'worked', he surmised that all he now needed was sufficient publicity. Where Ward was concerned, this was the easy part. He approached a number of well-known figures and began persuading them of the efficaciousness of his product. The writer Henry Fielding, who suffered from gout and dropsy (oedema), was highly impressed at the effect of the pill. Likewise Lord Chesterfield, the King's favourite minister, who not only supplied a glowing testimonial but also pressed Ward's product on all his friends, including George II. At the time, the King was suffering from 'a violent pain of the thumb'. This had been diagnosed as gout by the King's physician, the redoubtable Dr Richard Mead, who also happened to be President of the Royal College of Physicians. To the consternation of Dr Mead, Ward grasped the King's thumb…

Somehow, probably through purchase from an impecunious medical student, he came into the possession of recipes for the two medicines which would make him famous. These he called 'Ward's Pill and Drop'.

 and gave it so sudden a wrench, that the King cursed him and kicked his shins. Ward bore this very patiently and when the King was cool, respectfully asked him to move his thumb, which he did easily and found the pain gone.

Ward had gambled on his hunch that the King had merely dislocated his thumb.

Ward's fame and fortune were now guaranteed and he was soon using his powers of persuasion on the Lords of the Admiralty, convincing them that 'Ward's Pill and Drop' should be standard issue on every ship in the Royal Navy. However, Ward would eventually feel gratitude for the 'bounty he had been granted by fate', and used much of his fortune to endow no fewer than four London hospitals (which naturally all stocked large quantities of 'Ward's Pill and Drop').

Not all were impressed by Ward's ubiquitous pharmaceuticals. Queen Caroline demanded of the Duke of Marlborough whether it was true, as she had heard, that Ward's medicines had made a man mad.

'Yes, madam,' he replied, 'and his name is Mead.' The King's physician was to be further incensed when Ward decided to extend his range of products to include 'Ward's White Drop', 'a dropsy purging powder', and several other ingenious substances. This time Ward appears to have purchased his recipes from more talented practitioners and two of his new products would prove so successful (in strictly medical terms) that years later they would be granted the ultimate accolade of being included by the Royal College of Physicians in the *Pharmacopoeia Londinensis*. Fortunately, by this stage Mead was long dead, his bust staring stonily from his monument in Westminster Abbey. Ward himself was to be immortalised by the poet Alexander Pope, with the lines:

Of late, without the least pretence to skill,
Ward's grown a famed physician by a pill.

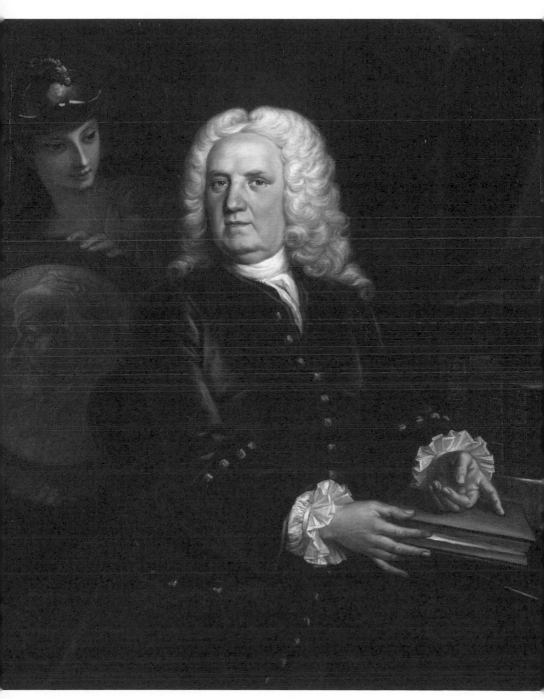

Richard Mead

'CHEVALIER' JOHN TAYLOR

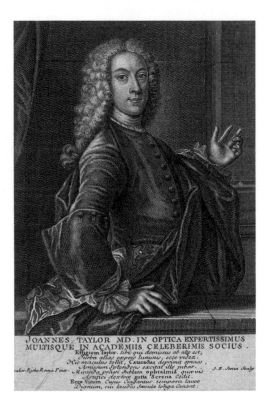

JOANNES TAYLOR MD. IN OPTICA EXPERTISSIMUS
MULTISQUE IN ACADEMIIS CELEBERIMIS SOCIUS.

'The eye is an angelic faculty. The eye in this respect is female. The eye is never tired of seeing and engaging with Nature's vigour.'

The third member of the trio in Hogarth's cartoon was 'Chevalier' John Taylor, who was quite the equal of Ward in self-promotion, but in actuality was a far more dangerous character. Indeed, he could be said to have represented just the kind of person that the Royal College of Physicians had been established to eliminate.

John Taylor was born in 1707, the son of a Norwich apothecary. In his youth he went to London to study under the pioneer surgeon and oculist William Cheselden, who would establish what later became the Royal College of Surgeons. At the time, the treating of diseases and afflictions of the human eye had barely emerged as a science. Indeed, Cheselden was responsible for a formative advance in ophthalmy. In 1728 he operated on a thirteen-year-old blind boy and succeeded in completely restoring his sight, by successfully removing the cataracts which had blighted his vision since birth. Throughout his life, Taylor would make a practice of trying to emulate this 'miraculous' operation, frequently with catastrophic effect.

According to Taylor himself in his autobiography, he showed great promise in his early studies – though others strongly doubt this. Either way, his ambitions far outran whatever talent he might have possessed. His career took off when at the age of twenty-six he set out to tour Europe as a travelling oculist, proclaiming his knowledge in the most extravagant (and often nonsensical) terms: 'The eye is an angelic faculty. The

ABOVE: 'Chevalier' John Taylor
OPPOSITE: The eye illustrated in William Cheselden's *Anatomy of the Human Body*, 1722

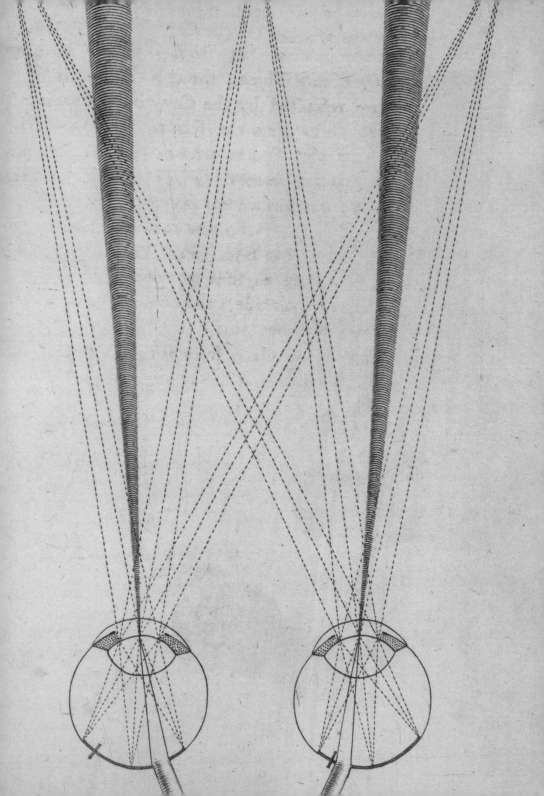

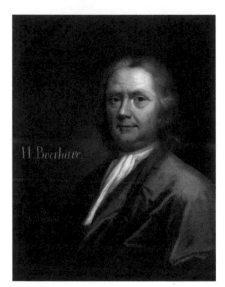

Dutch physician Herman Boerhaave

eye in this respect is female. The eye is never tired of seeing and engaging with Nature's vigour.' Like many a fine con-man, he appears to have been carried away by his rhetorical descriptions of his own talent. His travels would take him all over Europe, from Rome to Vienna, from Lisbon to Moscow. In the course of these journeys he attended many courts and claimed to have acquired many titles: 'Ophthalmiater Pontificator' to the Pope, 'Ophthalmiater Imperator' to the Holy Roman Emperor. 'Ophthalmiater Rex' to kings throughout the continent. Resemblances to his contemporary, the Baron von Münchhausen, may not be entirely coincidental.

However, in the course of these travels he also did irreparable harm. According to a modern authority, 'In Switzerland, he blinded hundreds of patients, he once confessed.' His treatment of Johan Sebastian Bach certainly didn't cure his eyesight and may well have contributed

to his death. On the other hand, Albrecht von Haller, the great Swiss 'father of modern physiology', referred to him as 'a skilful man, but too liberal of promises'.

Taylor returned to London in 1759, by now sporting the title 'chevalier' (a continental knighthood of suitably obscure provenance). He took up fashionable practice and treated George Frederic Handel with much the same effect as he had wreaked upon his fellow composer Bach. He began advertising himself as personal eye surgeon to George II, and gave public lectures where his rhetoric soared over the periwigged heads and powdered faces of his gullible audiences. On top of this, he always took care to emphasise his connections with the highest authorities (both medical and political). In his first book he modestly thanked Cheselden for the 'knowledge I have of this branch of medicine, such as it is'. Another was dedicated to the Royal College of Physicians of Edinburgh. Likewise he would frequently refer to his conversations, as if on equal terms, with the Dutch physician Herman Boerhaave, widely regarded as the finest medical mind in Europe. On the other hand, Dr Johnson regarded Taylor as 'the most ignorant man I ever knew'. The 'Chevalier' Taylor evidently did his best to steer clear of such forthright characters, which seems to have involved several hurried returns to the Continent. His silver tongue, and ability to be well down the road before anyone woke up to his misdeeds, also enabled him to acquire a reputation as a Casanova. And perhaps this would account for a certain mystery surrounding his death in 1772, probably in Rome. Ironically, by this time he himself had gone completely blind.

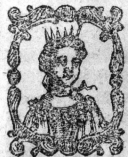

DAFFEY's ELIXIR Warehoufe,

AT the Maidenhead behind Bow Church in Cheapfide is fold for Two fhilings the Bottle, that admirable Cordial DAFFEY's ELIXIR SALUTIS, which is well known to exceed all the Medicines yet difcovered in chronical Difeafes, viz. Dropfy, Pryfick, Stone and Gravel Rheumatifm, Gout, Scurvy, Green Sicknefs, Cholick, King's-Evil, Confumption, Agues, and many other Difeafes incident to Men, Women and Children, which you may fee at large in the printed Directions. I need not fpeak in the Praife of this fafe and pleafant Cordial, it being well known throughout England, where it has been in great Ufe thefe fo Years.

N. B. It is, for the good of the Publick, truly and faihfully prepared of the choiceft Ingredients.

Advert for Dattey's (Daffy's) elixir (Wellcome Library, London)

A BAKER'S DOZEN OF ELIXIRS AND TINCTURES FOR ALL MANNER OF COMPLAINTS

Other lesser figures in this golden age include a variety of colourful miscreants, as well as their equally colourful medicines. These include the likes of Lunar Tincture, Daffy's Elixir, Elixir Magnum Stomachum, Mack's Anodyne Fluid, McLeod's Bread Pills (whose sole ingredient was bread), Rooke's Matchless Balsam, to say nothing of Choke Major and his 'Teething Necklace', Bromfield's Pilulae in Omnes Morbos (pills for all ills), as well as Samuel Solomon, whose spurious *Guide to Health* sold over 120,000 copies, spreading the word concerning his famous Balm of Gilead 'composed of the pure essence of virgin gold' (in fact, brandy and a few exotic herbs). Others were deluded by such phenomena as electrical medicines, to say nothing of the ever-popular gold medicines of all kinds and tinctures which purported to contain ground pearls or the like. All this conjures up a world of fly-by-nights and crooks hawking their more or less dangerous concoctions on street corners, or accompanied by snakes or dressed-up monkeys on rickety stages.

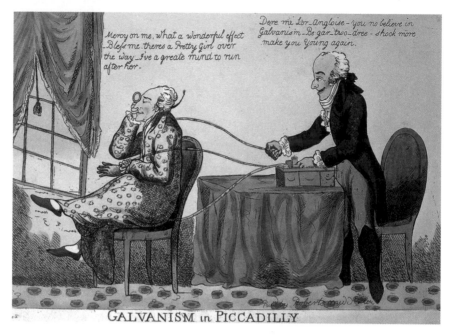

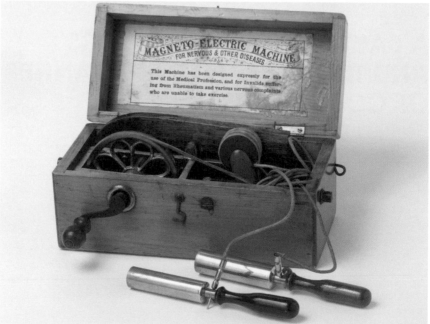

TOP: An affluent man receiving galvanic electric therapy from a French quack doctor (Wellcome Library, London)
ABOVE: A magneto-electric machine, late 19th century
OPPOSITE: Anthony Daffy's *Directions ... for taking ... elixir salutis*

DIRECTIONS

Given by mee

(ANTHONY DAFFY, Student in Physick.)

For taking my safe, innocent, and successful

CORDIAL DRINK;

CALLED

ELIXIR SALUTIS;

Proper to the Cure of each Distemper (in the Printed Sheet of its Virtues mentioned,) and suited unto the Patients several Ages, Sexes, and Constitutions.

The first general Observation.

FOR such persons as are opprest with *Chronical Distempers,* whether the *Gout, Stone, Collick, Ptissick, Dropsie,* &c. and have (divers Years) been tortured and bowed down under the burthen of them: I say, for Distempers habitual to, and seated in the Body; it cannot rationally be expected that this (or any Means under Heaven) may on a suddain effect their Cure, any more, than that a small shower of rain, (after a long season of Summers drought) should presently revive the parched and dying flowers and herbs of the field, and restore them

A   to

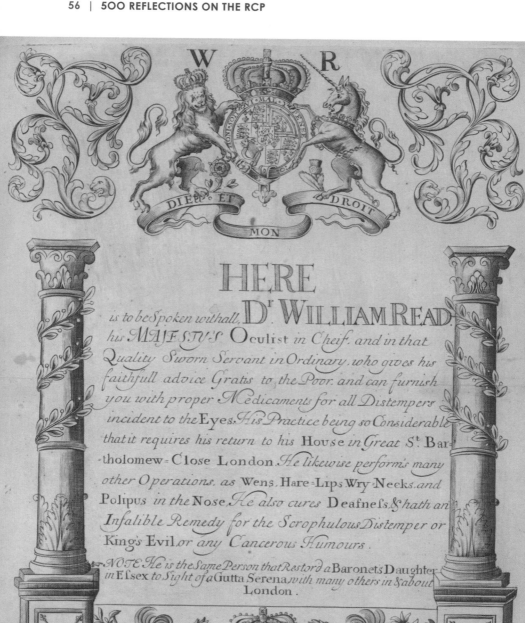

Advertisement for William Read (© Trustees of the British Museum)

WILLIAM READ

Yet not all such quacks and frauds were failures. Indeed, the jobbing haberdasher William Read, originally of Aberdeen, actually succeeded where the 'Chevalier' Taylor could only pretend, and got himself appointed royal oculist, in this case to Queen Anne. Having rehearsed his trade in Dublin, Read arrived in London with a glowing testimonial signed by a number of Irish worthies, including 'Narcissus (Lord Bishop of) Ferns'. Queen Anne suffered from poor eyesight and was constantly beset by quack oculists. But Read succeeded where the others failed – possibly through a degree of loquaciousness he had acquired during his time in Ireland. At any rate, he certainly went to great lengths to make sure that his name was known and his voice heard: according to Joseph Addison, essayist and founder of the *Spectator*, he was 'the most laborious advertiser of his time'. Be that as it may, Queen Anne was so enamoured of Read's abilities that she bestowed on him a knighthood. Whereupon he became 'a man of fashion, rich and ostentatious'. Guests to his dinner table were served 'his special brew of punch' in golden goblets. While his advertising bills, which so caught Addison's eye, spoke of his 'Medicaments for all Distempers incident to the Eyes…He likewise performs many other operations as Wens, Hare-Lips, Wry-Necks and Polipus in the Nose'. He even claimed to 'cure Deafness…the King's Evil or any Cancerous Humours'. A contemporary verse read:

The Queen, like Heav'n, shines equally on all,
Her favours now without distinction fall,
Great Read and slender Hannes, both knighted show,
That none their honours shall to merit owe.

Queen Anne was so enamoured of Read's abilities that she bestowed on him a knighthood. Whereupon he became 'a man of fashion, rich and ostentatious'.

The distinctionless exploits of 'slender' Hannes appear to have vanished into oblivion, a fate shared by the vast majority of Read's rival charlatans, who laboured so hard to have their quacking heard above the passing crowds. Once again, the Royal College remained unimpressed and, despite Read's knighthood, his royal appointment and his effusive testimonials, his inability to produce any certificate of medical qualification meant that he was repeatedly refused the licence he so coveted.

As Porter put it: 'Georgian public opinion was, of course, like everyone else, against quackery, but it did not always see eye-to-eye with the College as to who the quacks were'.

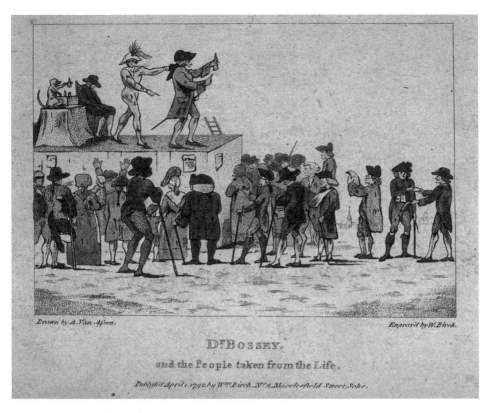

Drawn by A.Van Afsen.   Engravit by W.Birch.

DᴿBOSSEY.

and the People taken from the Life.

Publishit April 1.1792 by Wᴹ Birch.Nᵒ.2.Macclesfield Street.Soho.

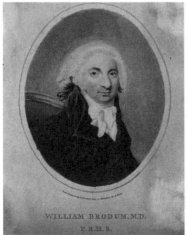

WILLIAM BRODUM, M.D.
F.R.H.S.

TOP: Dr Bossey Selling his wares (Wellcome Library, London)
ABOVE: Dr Brodum (Wellcome Library, London)

DR BRODUM

A case in point here is 'Dr' Brodum, who was of German-Jewish descent and began life as a footman to the celebrated Dr Bossey, a quack who had made himself a fortune performing cures on a stage he set up in Covent Garden, in a 'curative act' that included a large grey parrot. This must have inspired his footman, who branched out on his own to sell 'Nervous Cordial' and 'Botanical Syrup'. These nostrums were said to be 'a cure for the indiscretions of youth'. Brodum set up selling his wares from an address in Blackfriars, but made the mistake of installing outside his office a brass plate inscribed 'Dr Brodum', thus implying that he was a licensed physician. When word reached the Royal College of Physicians of this public outrage, Brodum was summoned to appear before the President and Censors of the College. Asked about his qualifications, Brodum produced a medical diploma from the Marischal College of Aberdeen. Since it was evident to the officers of the Royal College that Brodum had precious little knowledge of medical practice, he was asked how he had come by this certificate. Without batting an eyelid, Brodum replied that he had bought it, just like everyone else did. He even indicated that the certificate was signed by a Fellow of the Royal College. The President and Censors duly demanded that Brodum remove his brass plate, but when the 'doctor' refused to comply, the matter was dropped – presumably in order to avoid opening a can of worms.

JOANNA STEPHENS

Not all such brazen and successful quacks were men, as is evinced by the case of Mrs Joanna Stephens, who even in her lifetime was named 'the Queen of Quacks'. Mrs Stephens claimed to be 'the daughter of a Gentleman of good estate and family in Berkshire', and arrived on the London scene around 1735. She began advertising her own 'sovereign remedy' for The Stone (gallstones). During the period this was a widespread and painful disease, which was particularly prevalent among the upper classes. Mrs Stephens' cure soon began attracting peers of the realm, bishops and even duchesses; and initially a number of her clients were persuaded – or persuaded themselves – that her 'stone-dissolving' medicament relieved them of their symptoms. However, not all were so persuaded and after three years Mrs Stephens decided to cash in on her luck, and her 'sovereign remedy', by selling its secret to the nation. In April 1738 an announcement appeared in the *Gentleman's Magazine*:

> **Mrs Stephens has proposed to make her medicine publick on Consideration of £5,000 to be raised by contribution, and lodged with Mr Drummond, Banker; he has received since the eleventh of this month about £500 on that account.**

Five thousand pounds was a colossal sum: more than enough to buy a large house and estate in the country. Mrs Stephens' publick subscription succeeded in raising £1,356 – much of it from the worthies who considered themselves cured by her secret remedy. The Earl of Godolphin even contributed £100. But Mrs Stephens chose to hold out for the full amount before divulging her secret. Whereupon her influential friends decided to petition Parliament, so that her 'sovereign remedy' could be purchased by the nation. A committee was set up to enquire into the efficacy of Mrs Stephens' cure. This included several lords, members of Parliament and the noted philosopher–physician Dr David Harley. When Dr Harley revealed that he himself had been cured by Mrs Stephens, the committee decided in her favour and she was duly awarded enough to buy her country seat. The contents of the powder were then published in the *Gentleman's Magazine*:

3 *per C.* Ann. 105 ¼	Died under 2 Years old ---	808	
Bank 142 ½	Between 2 and 5 ----	204	
—— Circul. 25 : Pre.	Between 5 and 10 ----	66	
Mil. Bank 120	Between 10 and 20 ----	64	
India 173	Between 20 and 30 ----	109	
—Bonds 6*l.* 14*s.*	Between 30 and 40 ----	155	
African 14	Between 40 and 50 ----	164	
Royal Aff. 107 ½	Between 50 and 60 ----	134	
Lon. ditto 14	Between 60 and 70 ----	107	
5 *p. C.* Em. Loan 100	Between 70 and 80 ----	79	
7 *p. C.* Ditto 111	Between 80 and 90 ----	36	
English Cop. 3*l.* 5*s.*	Between 90 and 100 ----	12	
Welfh ditto 15*s.*			

Weekly Burials.

Oct.. 3. — 376
10. — 534
17. — 523
24. — 505
—————
1938

S. S. old Annuities Divid. 2 *pr Ct*, pay the 23d *London* Affurance Divid. 6 *s.* per Share.   1938

Peck Loaf, Wheaten—21 d.
Wheat 26 *s.* per *Quar.*
Hay per load 50*s.*
Beft Hops 3*l.* 15*s.*
Coals 25*s.* per Chaldron as fet by the Lord Mayor and Aldermen, purfuant to the new Act.

ACCOUNT *of Perfons who have taken* Mrs STEPHENS's *Medicines for the* STONE.

THE following is a Copy, of fuch Accounts as have been fent to Mr *Harding* on the Pavement in St *Martins Lane*, in compliance with Mrs *Stephens*'s requeft, the Originals of which may be feen there, by any one who defires it.

I have prefixed a fhort Extract from the ten Cafes which I printed laft *March*, and fhall continue to furnifh the Public with all the Information I can concerning this Matter. For which purpofe I humbly entreat all Perfons who have formerly taken thefe Medicines, or who do fo now, whether they have received Benefit or Mifchief, a perfect Cure or only Relief from their Complaints, to fend in their Cafes to Mr *Harding*, and to be as particular as they can confiftently with Brevity. Thofe who have received Benefit cannot deny fo reafonable a Favour to Mrs *Stephens*, but Juftice to Mankind equally obliges all to publifh the real Effects of Medicines which pretend to be fo important : Nor ought fmall Difficulties to hinder any one from complying with an Obligation of fuch a Nature.

The Contribution is advanced to about 1250*l.* a particular Account of which fhall be printed fhortly. In the mean time I beg leave to interceed with the Public for the Miferable : If thefe Medicines fhould prove ineffectual, it is fome Charity even to undeceive thofe unhappy Perfons who neglect better Methods from the falfe Hopes afforded by them. But if they fhould prove effectual, let every good Man think how glad he will be to have contributed to and haftened their Publication ; and where there are fuch Judges, with fo ftrict, open and impartial a Method of Trial propofed, as that of the Hofpitals, it is certain that Mrs *Stephens* cannot have the Reward unlefs fhe deferves it.

October 14, 1738.   D. *Hartley.*

A fhort EXTRACT from the ten CASES.

1. The Right Rev. the Lord Bifhop of *Bath* and *Wells*, had the Symptoms of a Stone in the left Kidney, took Mrs *Stephens*'s Medicines, voided many fmall Flakes and Fragments of Stone in a foft State, became very eafy and able to ride, or go in a Coach without Inconvenience.

2. Mr *Binford* of *Exeter*, had the Symptoms of a Stone in the Bladder, was examined twice by Mr *Patch*, an eminent Surgeon there, with the Finger in Ano, who felt a large Stone both times ; he took the Medicines, voided much brown Grit, many thin Scales, many thick Shells, confifting of different Coats, and fome folid pieces of Stone, and became free from all his Complaints ; Mr *Patch* after this examined him again with the Finger in Ano, but could not find any Stone.

3. Mr *Botton* of *Newcaftle upon Tyne*, had the Symptoms of a Stone in the Bladder for about two Years attended with violent Pains. He took the Medicines for about five Months, they increafed his Pains a little for the firft two Months, afterwards he grew much eafier and was at laft quite freed from them. He voided many Pieces and one entire Stone weighing about 5 Grains.

4. The Hon. Mr *Carteret*, Poft-Mafter General, had the Symptoms of a Stone in the Bladder, took the Medicines, voided many Pieces of Stone, with a Kernel, and became free from all his Complaints.

5. Mr *Daubuz* in *Throgmorton Street*, had the Symptoms of a Stone in the Bladder, took the Medicines, voided three fmall Stones, and became perfectly well.

6. Mr *Snape* in *Panton Street*, had the Symptoms of a Stone in the Bladder, took the Medicines, voided many pieces of Stone in a foft State, and became perfectly well.

7. The Rev. Dr *Sykes* in *Great Marlborough Street*

The Pills consist of Snails calcined, wild carrott seeds, burdock seeds, ashen keys, hips and hawes – all burnt to blackness – Alicant soap and honey.

A veritable witch's brew, if ever there was one. And immediately upon receiving her money Mrs Stephens vanished from the scene. This story had a sad coda: despite having been 'cured' of The Stone, Harley would die of this malady some years later.

WILLIAM BUCHAN AND JOHN THEOBALD

Dr Harley was not the only member of his profession to be taken in by quacks. Several genuine, licensed practitioners had begun publishing medical works, ranging from pamphlets to lengthy volumes, intended for the general public. In the main, these described various diseases, their symptoms and so forth, and then detailed which were the best medicines to take for their treatment. These were 'aimed at a health-conscious lay readership' and soon began selling in their thousands. Indeed, it was said of William Buchan's *Domestic Medicine*, published in 1789, that 'every Scottish cottage had a copy of Buchan and the Bible'. Less reputable publications were quick to follow. John Theobald's *Every Man his Own Physician* included Joanna Stephens's cure for The Stone. Others descended into pure fiction, to such an extent that the poet laureate Robert Southey suggested such works should be entitled 'Every Man His Own Poisoner'.

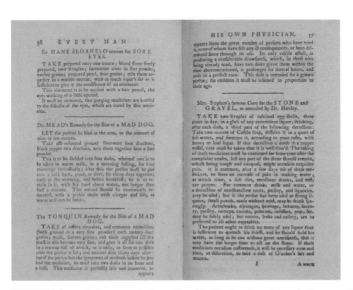

OPPOSITE: Account of persons who have taken Mrs Stephens's medicines for the stone, *Gentlemen's Magazine*, October 1738

ABOVE: Mrs Stephens's cure for the stone and gravel in John Theobold's *Every Man His Own Physician*, 1766

Ex libris Societatis Med Offic Alhed
Dom Gul Saunders M.D

Encomium Argenti Vivi:

A

TREATISE

UPON THE

USE and PROPERTIES

OF

QUICKSILVER;

OR,

The Natural, Chymical, and Physical History of that surprising MINERAL, extracted from the Writings of the best Naturalists, Chymists, and Physicians.

Wherein its various Operations are accounted for, and the Use of it recommended.

WITH

Some REMARKS upon the Animadversions of Dr. TURNER upon BELLOSTE.

By a Gentleman of *Trinity College Cambridge.*

LONDON:

Printed for STEPHEN AUSTEN in St. *Paul's* Church *Yard*, and sold by *J. Roberts* in *Warwick-Lane.*

THOMAS DOVER (DR QUICKSILVER)

Many qualified doctors could, in their own right, prove a danger to their patients. One such was Dr Thomas Dover who, at the age of twenty-seven, received a medical degree from Cambridge in 1687 and then studied in London under no less than Thomas Sydenham, known as 'the father of English medicine'. Dover then set up practice in the port of Bristol, at this time the second-richest city in England, where he earned a small fortune. Yet he soon observed that even larger fortunes were being made in the city out of privateering expeditions (little more than licensed piracy against Spanish treasure-bearing ships en route from South America to Spain). After investing his money with one such expedition mounted by one of his sea captain patients, 'Captain' Dover set off with his friend on a remarkable series of adventures. Just one of these will have to suffice: while sailing in the Pacific, Dover's ship noticed a light on the remote Juan Fernandez Island and put ashore to discover the shipwrecked Thomas Selkirk (who would become the model for Defoe's *Robinson Crusoe*). After nearly twenty years of travels and adventures, Dover returned to Bristol a very rich man, but quickly lost his £6,000 fortune in the South Sea Bubble. By now he was in his sixties and he decided to return to medicine. To re-establish himself as a physician, he applied for a licence from the Royal College of Physicians, but he appeared to have forgotten most of his medicine and was lucky to scrape through the exams. He returned to private practice, but his opinionated and irascible bedside manner, especially concerning modern treatments that had become popular during his absence, ensured he earned little money. So to recoup his fortunes he decided to write a popular medical book, which he called *The Ancient Physician's Legacy to his Country*. According to his biographer R. S. Morton and others, this book 'shows some degree of wisdom regarding pharmacology, his knowledge of medicine is…. small, while his descriptions of some diseases are presented in the "flimsiest fashion" and "outrageous inaccuracies are set down with no little dogmatism".' He also used the opportunity to accuse the Royal College of Physicians of prejudice, his colleagues of bias against him, and to complain about the lamentable state of contemporary medicine. At one point he recommended 'crude mercury' as a cure for syphilis – a widespread but dangerous prescription. But this was not enough for Dover. His most persistent and notorious recommendation was that quicksilver (mercury) was in fact a cure for all manner of diseases – when, as is well known (and was well known at the time), ingestion of this poisonous substance was liable to prove extremely harmful, if not lethal. Dover's *Legacy* went into innumerable editions and was even translated, gaining for him the popular nickname 'Dr Quicksilver'. Twenty years after his death in 1742, editions of his *Legacy* were still being published and its recommendations followed. Southey had but the half of it: patients might poison themselves following the advice of quacks, but licensed doctors were capable of doing this too.

JAMES GRAHAM

Syphilis was not the only widespread sexual complaint of the period, and the quack sexologist James Graham struck a particularly lucrative seam when he promised his clients that he could cure them of all sexual ills and restore them to their utmost vigour and fecundity. This was precisely what the public wanted to hear and Graham was only too willing to relieve them of their money in providing his service. The extravagance of his claims was only matched by the extravagant performances of his public lectures and his extravagant charges.

Graham had been born in Edinburgh in 1745, the son of a sadler. Despite such lowly circumstances, he benefitted from the superior Scottish education of the period and ended up studying medicine – but failed to finish the course. Regardless of this oversight, he then travelled south of the border and set up a medical practice in Yorkshire. Some years later he married, but soon found it expedient to set sail for America. Here he met Benjamin Franklin, who introduced him to the wonders of electricity. Graham quickly adopted this 'magical force' to medical use. He constructed a 'Celestial Bed', where electricity, magnetism and music were to be harnessed to such effect that 'Children of the most perfect beauty could be begotten'. Forced to flee the American Revolution, he returned to England, now convinced by his new invention that he was 'a man of destiny'. To begin with he set up practice in Bath, where his new 'electrical' cures soon began attracting society patients such as Georgiana, Duchess of Devonshire. 1780 found him in London, where he opened a sumptuously decorated 'Temple of Health'. Here he gave lectures to a paying public of society beaus and their ladies in the Great Hall, whose walls were covered with the crutches, spectacles and ear trumpets of patients he had cured. Afterwards he would sell such medicines as his 'Electrical Aether', 'Elixir of Life' and 'Nervous Aetherial'. The central feature of his new establishment was The Grand Celestial Bed, which could be hired for £50 a night. The Temple of Health soon became one of the sights of London, with society audiences and distinguished foreign visitors cramming his ever more spectacular lectures. These featured his celebrated 'Goddesses of Health': flimsily clad young women who paraded the stage as 'models of physical perfection'. His performances and general behaviour became more and more extravagant, the more he felt that he was fulfilling his destiny. Porter describes how 'aided by a bevy of lightly-clad "goddesses of health", he championed

Syphilis was not the only widespread sexual complaint of the period, and the quack sexologist James Graham struck a particularly lucrative seam when he promised his clients that he could cure them of all sexual ills and restore them to their utmost vigour and fecundity.

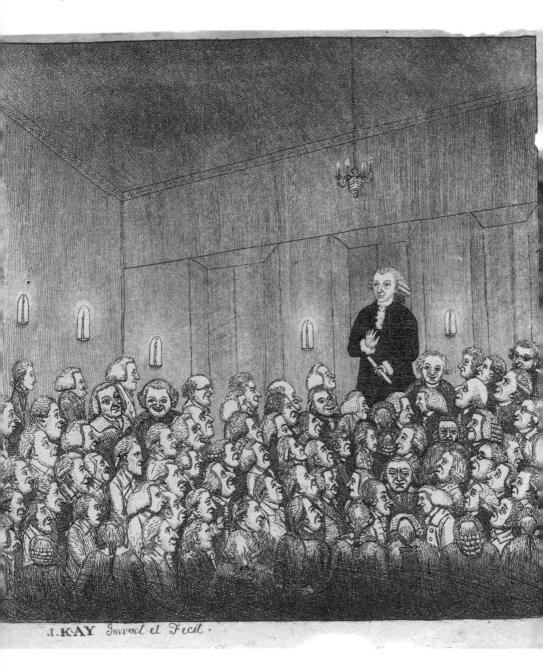

J.KAY Invent et Fecit.

James Graham addressing a crowd

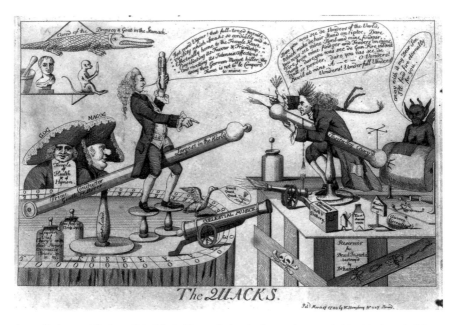

James Graham and Gustavus Katerfelto battling against each other, each surrounded by objects symbolising his practice (Wellcome Library, London)

the omni-curative properties of mud-baths and had himself repeatedly buried fakir-like,[4] naked, for days on end, fasting all the while'. Graham claimed that for this ritual 'fresh, icy, cold earth brought from the top of Hampstead Hill' was preferable. Though for those too busy to acquire such material and undergo the entire lengthy process 'even a turf strapped to the chest…was better than nothing'.

 With money rolling in, 1781 saw the opening in fashionable Pall Mall of a second premises, which he called 'The Temple of Hymen'. But by this stage his extravagance had overreached itself and he fell heavily into debt. He soon left for Edinburgh, where the contents of his 'aetherial lectures' so outraged the less tolerant Scottish authorities that he was flung into jail. His fall from grace appears to have finally upset the precarious balance of his mind. According to Southey, 'Graham was half mad and his madness finally got the better of his knavery. He would madden himself with ether, run out into the streets and strip himself to clothe the first beggar he met'. He attempted to found a new religion and then embarked upon a succession of fasting exploits aimed at prolonging his life. Both of these enterprises failed and he died in 1794 at the age of forty-nine.

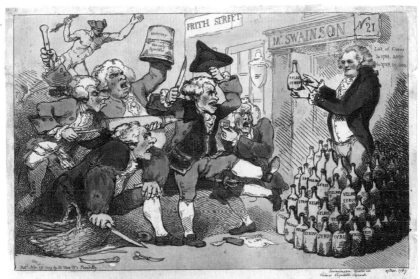

MERCURY and his ADVOCATES DEFEATED, or VEGETABLE INTRENCHMENT

Isaac Swainson demonstrates the virtues of Velnos syrup outside his house (© Trustees of the British Museum)

ISAAC SWAINSON AND DR MERCIER

Graham was not the only notable quack who exploited the sexual anxieties of the Georgian age. Isaac Swainson was born in Lancashire in 1746 and began life as a woollen draper, but decided to head south to London to make his fortune. Here he found employment as an assistant to a Dr Mercier, a physician of Huguenot descent who had set up practice in Soho. When Dr Mercier retired he sold his assistant a herbal remedy which had been concocted by a somewhat elusive character called Vergery de Velnos. Swainson embarked upon an advertising campaign for 'Velnos' Vegetable Syrup', claiming that this patent preparation could cure all venereal diseases – including 'the pox', 'the French Disease' and 'The Clape'. He even wrote a small sixteen-page booklet instructing patients how to take this medicine. 'Persons of strong habits and tenacious bowels may begin with two or three spoonfuls night and morning'. In a period when many were suffering the painful and poisonous mercury cure for venereal disease, Venlos' Vegetable Syrup soon proved a highly popular substitute. For good measure, Swainson also claimed that his vegetable syrup could cure 'leprosy, gout, scrophula, dropsy, small pox, consumption, tape worms, cancer, scurvy and diarrhoea'. As a result, Swainson was soon selling 20,000 bottles of the

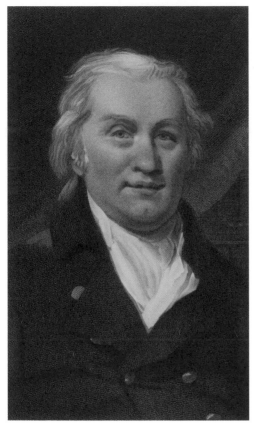

Isaac Swainson

Swainson became such an authority on botany that he would in time be honoured by having a plant named after him. This is the variety of desert pea now known as *Swansonia formosa*, which would later be adopted as the emblem of South Australia.

By all accounts, Swainson became a popular local figure, renowned in Twickenham for riding his coach and horses full gallop out through the monumental gates of his new home, where he lived to the venerable age of sixty-six – having been 'enriched by vegetables and immortalised by a plant'.

BISHOP BERKELEY'S TAR WATER

syrup a year, bringing him an income of £5,000. Upon making his fortune, Swainson invested in a mansion set amid its own extensive grounds in Twickenham, on the south-west outskirts of London. Here he transformed himself from a quack into a genuine scientist, laying out botanical gardens which contained all manner of genuine medicinal herbs. He also appears to have studied genuine medicine during this period, but upon gaining an MD he was not able to obtain a licence from the Royal College of Physicians on account of his previous incarnation. However,

However, not all quacks were fortune-hunters of questionable motive. Few could have a more blameless reputation than Bishop George Berkeley, who together with John Locke is now recognised as one of the pioneers of Empiricism. This philosophy insisted that all we can know for certain must be based upon experience. Berkeley was possessed of exceptional intellectual penetration, capable of pursuing ideas to their logical limits. He alone was able to detect the logical fault in Newton's conception of calculus. And such was Berkeley's philosophical penetration that he saw through the materialism which others supposed to be the ultimate conclusion of Locke's Empiricism. According to Berkeley, all that we experience are sensations – which we only view as material objects because our minds form these perceptions into the false idea of a persistent material reality. Therefore, when I do not perceive the world, it does not in fact exist. However, his *reductio ad absurdum* of empirical thinking did not affect the way he lived. After crossing the Atlantic (which must have vanished when he was asleep), he lived for several years in America. Here he wrote the poem which gave rise to 'Westward ho!', with the result that the University of California at Berkeley is now named after him. After returning from America he lived in the small, remote Irish city of Cloyne, of which he became bishop. Here he published *Siris: a chain of philosophical reflexions and enquiries concerning the virtues of tar water.* In this he extolled the virtues of drinking a solution of pine tar in water as a cure for all ills. Pine tar had been used for centuries as a disinfectant, but for Berkeley it was something more:

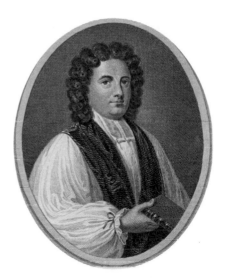

> **Hail vulgar juice of never-fading pine!**
> **Cheap as thou art, thy virtues are divine.**

It is difficult to conceive of how one of the finest intellects of his age could have been taken in by such nonsense. And had it been just the whim of an ageing bishop, this might not have mattered. But when Berkeley published his work on tar water in 1744, it outsold all of his other works and soon became the panacea of the age. Fielding tried it for his dropsy, but it didn't work; later, its popularity would revive in the Victorian era, when Dickens would refer to its disgusting taste in *Great Expectations*.

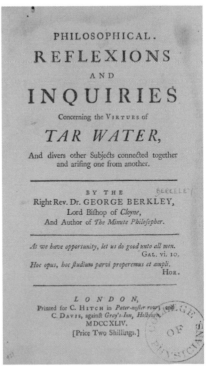

TOP: George Berkeley
ABOVE: Title page of Berkeley's *Philosophical Reflections ...*, 1744

JOHN LOCKE'S SILVER TUBE

This brings us to the curious case of Berkeley's philosophical predecessor John Locke. A man of many parts, Locke not only founded Empiricism but also had original ideas on a wide range of topics, including economics (he became a commissioner for trade) and political liberty (his principles would be incorporated into the American constitution).

Less well known is his study of medicine, much of which was conducted alongside his lifelong Oxford friend, the great Thomas Sydenham. But according to Locke's biographer Fox Bourne, Locke chose to study medicine 'in his own way, and not in accordance with university rules'. Admittedly, 'The teaching… was nearly as useless in the education of competent doctors as were Latin verse-writing and Aristotelian disputation in the education of useful politicians.' (Shades of the pair of Oxford 'doctors' who turned up at Cambridge and were deemed to be 'illiterate'.) Even so, Locke's case is strange. 'The Oxford requirements as regards medical education were so slight, that it is not easy to understand why he should have failed to comply with these'. Despite such lack of qualification, Locke was perfectly prepared to take up the post of personal physician to his friend Lord Ashley, who was at the time a close friend of Charles II and the most

influential politician in the land. Ashley had long suffered from an agonising internal malady, which Locke diagnosed as a suppurating cyst of the liver. Despite his complete lack of experience or qualification, Locke then carried out an operation which involved inserting into Ashley's abdomen a silver tube, the purpose of which was to drain the fluid from the abscess. Amazingly, this proved successful. Locke then found himself faced with a quandary. Should he leave the tube permanently inserted (and risk infection) or should he remove the tube (and risk his friend dying of 'a new depositing of poison in the abdomen'). According to Fox Bourne, 'Locke sent a sort of circular, inviting opinions on this point'. Locke himself made it clear to his expert medical advisers that he believed the silver tube should remain. Sydenham and others agreed with him and the silver tube stayed put. 'Satirists afterwards made great fun of Lord Ashley's silver tube, but the silver tube kept him alive to hear this satire'.

There appears to have been more than a little professional jealousy among the leading experts whom Locke consulted. As Bourne explains: 'Thomas Sydenham, a physician infinitely superior to them all, [was] then, and for some time after, looked upon by most other doctors, and by the great mass of the public who followed their lead, as little better

'Satirists afterwards made great fun of Lord Ashley's silver tube, but the silver tube kept him alive to hear this satire'.

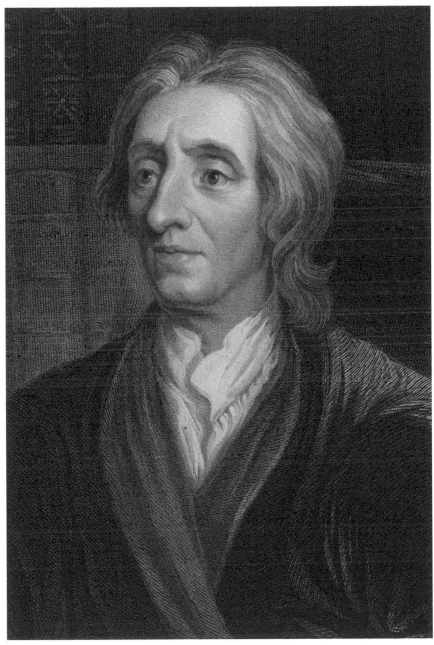

John Locke

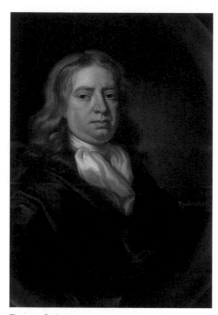

Thomas Sydenham

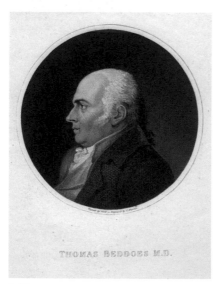

Dr Thomas Beddoes

than a quack'. As 'Harvey the circulator' had discovered, even the finest minds and practitioners in the land were not immune from accusations of quackery. And on this occasion, the enemies of Thomas Sydenham had a point: despite his transcendent reputation at Oxford as the 'English Hippocrates', he too had seen no reason to graduate as an MD.[5]

THOMAS BEDDOES

As far as genuine quacks were concerned, these now found themselves facing a formidable adversary in the form of Dr Thomas Beddoes, whom Porter christened the 'Grand Inquisitor of the Quacks'. Beddoes was born in Bristol in 1760. From the outset, he proved to be a man of formidable temperament and even more formidable intellect. At Oxford he studied French, German and Spanish, alongside the usual Ancient Greek and Latin, before moving on to Edinburgh to study medicine. Here he gained a reputation for cantankerous behaviour, especially with regard to his theory that modern medicine required a modern chemical foundation. In pursuit of this idea he travelled to Paris to meet the great French chemist Antoine Lavoisier, whose chemical ideas confirmed him in his beliefs, but whose anti-Revolutionary ideas he found most distressing. He then returned to Oxford, where his original ideas attracted few defenders, but his angry lectures proved highly popular drama with the students of the day. In his spare time he would track down quacks and go to great pains to ensure that they faced the full force of the law. In 1793 he finally left Oxford, 'with a reputation for being a short (and short tempered) radical'. In 1801 he set up practice in London, 'despairing of the ideas of the rich and the poor', contracted an unhappy marriage, and devoted the majority of his time to the campaign for which he will always be remembered. Previously, his persecution of quacks had been more of a hobby, but this now developed into a full-blown mania as he sought out hapless malpractitioners wherever he could find them, ensuring that they were quickly removed to Newgate prison. Unfortunately his irascible and melancholic temperament eventually got the better of him and in 1808, at the age of forty-eight, he committed suicide.

JOHN COAKLEY LETTSOM

More mild-mannered in his pursuit of quackery was the London physician John Coakley Lettsom, whose particular pet hate was the practice of 'piddle-tasting', a distasteful and largely ineffective method designed for the most part to impress upon patients the dedication to which their physicians were willing to go in order to diagnose their illness. Since earliest times physicians had considered the analysis (mostly by taste) of a patient's urine as an important diagnostic method. Lettsom's *bête noire* was Theodor Mysersbach, a German practitioner of the art of 'urine casting', as it was known. Lettsom's persistent attacks on Myersbach and his methods would lead to the near-extinction of this practice.

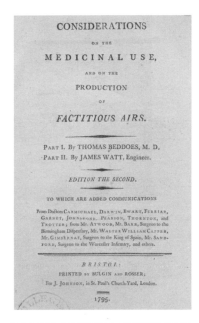

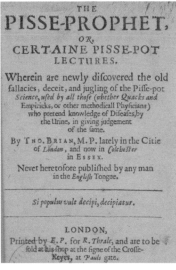

TOP: Title page of Thomas Beddoes and James Watt's *Considerations on the Medicinal Use … of Factitious Airs*, 1795
ABOVE: Title page of Thomas Brian's *The Pisse-Prophet*, 1637. A century before Lettsom, Brian had opposed those who abused the examination of urine which in the 17th century was used to advise on marriage and tell fortunes

RESTORES THE HAIR.

PROMOTES THE GROWTH

ARRESTS THE FALL.

STRENGTHENS THE ROOT

WITHOUT A RIVAL.

HEALTH TO

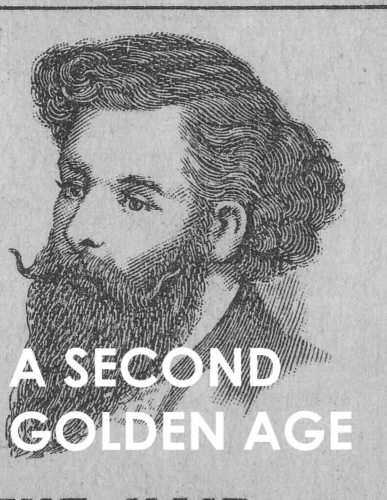

Such was the widespread craving among the populace to believe they could be cured – of what ills they had, or could be convinced they had – that the Golden Age of eighteenth-century quackery quickly gave way to the Golden Age of nineteenth-century quackery. This would prove little more plausible in its manifestations, despite its more modern appeal to 'Enlightenment', an element which had often been lacking among earlier practitioners. Instead of lively and intriguing crowd-pullers such as dressed-up pet monkeys playing drums, squawking parrots, rows of brightly coloured canaries with little bells and the like, the modern quack was more likely to present himself (or herself) as a person of reason, appealing to 'the scientific method'. Yet the practitioners, and their clients, remained for the most part inspired by a similarly misguided optimism. As such they were just as liable to find themselves hauled before the Censors of the Royal College of Physicians. However, by this time the power of the College had been considerably reduced, with much of its jurisdiction being sequestrated by the law and other professional medical bodies. Like the apothecaries, the surgeons and barber-surgeons had long-standing disputes with the Royal College of Physicians.

Even so, a summons to appear before the Censors of the Royal College of Physicians was no light matter. Throughout its several changes of venue, the buildings housing the Royal College have always placed great emphasis on the Censors' Room. To this day, this inner sanctum retains the Spanish Oak panelling which was such an imposing feature of the eighteenth-century Censors' Room at Warwick Lane. As in the days of yore, the miscreant summoned to appear would find himself standing before a formidable array of powerful figures. At least six Censors would be seated around the large polished oval

PREVIOUS PAGE: Part of an advert for Edwards' 'Harlene' for the hair (Wellcome Library, London)
BELOW: A meeting in the Long Room of the College's Warwick Lane building. The oak panelling can be seen

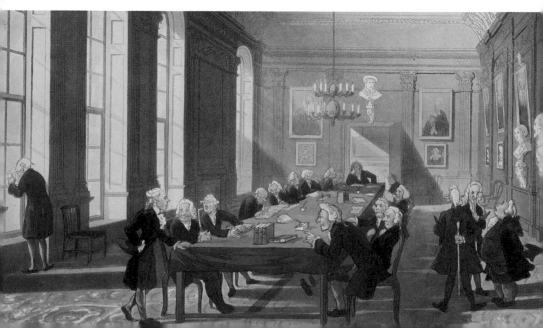

table before him, with the chairman's position at the head of the table almost always occupied by the President of the College himself. Beneath the austere gaze of the portraits lining the panelled walls – previous presidents, fellows, celebrated medical grandees – the intimidated defendant would be expected to plead his case with due deference. And woe betide the man (or woman) who incautiously chose to insist upon their innocence without a display of sufficient respect for his judges. Despite the austere and formal surroundings, the interrogation suffered by the defendant was not always limited to the niceties expected of such a solemn judicial court. Official proceedings were liable to degenerate into less decorous occasions. Outraged bewigged Censors frequently rose from their seats to approach and berate the defendant, shouting directly into his face, with no restraint upon the opinion of his heinous deeds and unspeakable character, sometimes even pushing him back against the panelled wall. On the other hand, actual physical violence was usually avoided out of deference to the chairman's calls for order. The authority of the chairman was for the most part absolute, with his verdict often decided by his first sight of the defendant as he entered the room. (Or, in some of the more publicised cases, before even then.)

Such was the widespread craving among the populace to believe they could be cured – of what ills they had, or could be convinced they had – that the Golden Age of eighteenth-century quackery quickly gave way to the Golden Age of nineteenth-century quackery.

The Censors' Room in the College's St Andrews Place building with the oak panelling from Warwick Lane

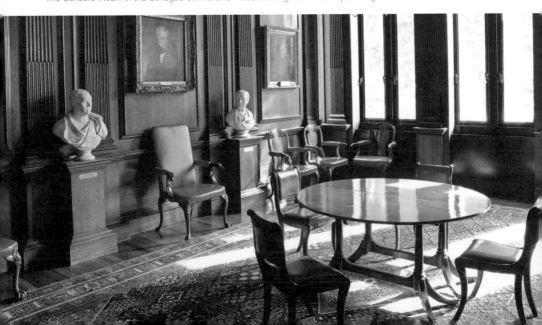

ARTHUR POINTING AND HIS ORIENTAL TOILET COMPANY

Despite such sanctions, ever more ingenious quacks now began to proliferate in the new scientific era of the second golden age. An early example of this new breed is perhaps best epitomised by the case of Arthur Pointing. Despite his enlightened veneer, his claims and his optimism remained as outrageous as ever. Indeed, one of his earliest ventures was a scheme 'to convince short people that he could make them taller' – an unlikely enterprise which proved to be his first great success.

Pointing had been born in 1867 in the fashionable London suburb of Stoke Newington, renowned during the period for its private boarding schools catering for foreign pupils. (Both the young German philosopher Arthur Schopenhauer and the American poet Edgar Allan Poe were educated here.) Pointing's initial uplifting venture was accompanied by adverts which asked: 'Are you little?' and went on to recommend his 'invisible elevators' which could be supplied by 'The Oriental Toilet Company' of 77 Strand.[6] Within three months he had made £300 (when a labourer earned less than £2 a week). But, in the words of a modern expert in this field, Caroline Rance: 'By this time, however, enough people had also realized that they were still as short as ever'. Pointing was arrested and his trial at the Old Bailey attracted an angry crowd of people of limited stature. Pointing escaped on a technicality: the judge ruled that the Oriental Toilet Company was a legitimate business.

Pointing decided to try his luck elsewhere and took ship for America, where he joined the Yukon Gold Rush. He returned, goldless, some years later. But while crossing the United States his eyes had been opened by the snake oil salesmen and their ilk. He began collecting their hand-bills and on his return to England began mimicking their 'brash confidence and outrageous claims', as well as their mock-scientific and informative style.

POINTING'S ANTIDIPSO

Inspired by several patent medicines, Pointing came up with the idea of 'Antidipso', a cure for alcoholism containing 'an obscure tropical plant [that] expels the alcoholic poison'. (Its strong purgative nature lent at least an element of truth to this claim.) According to an accompanying booklet, *Bright Beams of Hope*, this plant had been discovered in South America by an (unnamed) English physician and had subsequently been acquired by the Ward Chemical Company – a name that consciously harked back to the great Joshua 'Spot' Ward of 'pill and drop' fame.[7]

Where Antidipso was concerned, Pointing's great insight was that while most drunkards were not always interested in curing themselves, their wives were. His bold American-style advertisement and accompanying booklets were specifically addressed to women, assuring them that Antidipso 'can be given in Tea, Coffee or Food, thus absolutely and secretly Curing the Patient in a Short Time without his knowledge'. Bearing this in mind, Pointing produced two different colours of Antidipso, which could be secretly administered according to the colour of the food or drink the unwitting patient was consuming. And to add the final touch, Pointing's booklets boasted a reproduction of 'a certificate of medical excellence' from A. B. Griffiths, 'Principal of the Brixton School of Pharmacy'. Griffiths was a character who graced the fringes of the medical scene and his name appears on many products during this period. For one guinea (just over £1), he was willing to issue a certificate testifying to the 'marked therapeutic action' of any product placed before him.

When medical authorities tested Pointing's product it was found to contain around 80 per cent milk sugar and 20 per cent potassium bromide. There was no sign of any herb, South American or otherwise. However, such authorities as the Royal College of Physicians were faced with a quandary. If taken in sufficiently large quantities, Antidipso was liable to induce nausea and diarrhoea – thus voiding the digestive tract of any alcoholic content. On the other hand, in small doses it would have no effect at all (not even a placebo effect, as the patient would be unaware of having taken the medicine). On what grounds was Antidipso to be banned? The *Lancet* expressed its anger: 'To raise false hopes in those whose lot it is to be tied to a drunkard is disgraceful and no punishment can be too bad for the person who profits by such deceit.' But no action was taken.

It was soon clear that Pointing was raking in the profits. Two packets of Antidipso, each containing four dozen sachets of powder, could be purchased for £1. The ingredients they contained cost a couple of pence at most. Meanwhile the Ward Chemical Company went from strength to strength and Pointing was able to open sumptuous offices in prestigious Regent Street. Alas, he did not live long enough to enjoy the full fruits of his success. At the age of thirty-seven he was suddenly felled by the hideous effects of tertiary syphilis, a disease which he had probably contracted in the same American West where he discovered the secret of his success among the bold claims and outrageous patter of the snake oil salesmen. A year later, in 1910, Pointing was dead, leaving a fortune of almost £39,000.

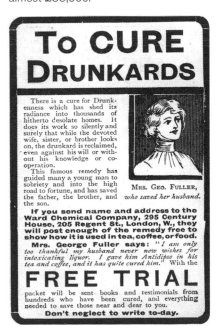

Advert for Antidipso

WONDER MEDICINES: BALDNESS, FATNESS, ALLAN'S ANTI-FAT, BLADDERWRACK, FIGUROIDS

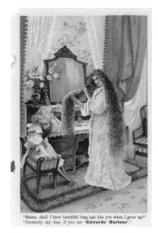

"Mama, shall I have beautiful long hair like you when I grow up?"
"Certainly, my dear, if you use 'Edwards' Harlene'."

Advertisement for Edwards' Harlene (Wellcome Library, London)

Quackery in the new golden age took a more specific approach. Panaceas and cure-all 'wonder medicines' did not entirely vanish from the scene, but they no longer dominated it. The scatter-gun approach gave way to more selective targets. Specific, but perennial complaints – such as shortness – now began to attract the attention of the modern quack. Alongside the ever-present alcoholism and baldness, another widespread complaint was 'fatness'. Then, as now, adverts disguised as articles appeared in the popular press asking, 'Is Fatness a Social Offence?' The *Daily Mail* declared: 'The fat woman is an enemy to the artistic uplift, for she is entirely too heavy for any wings of fancy to raise.' Such suggestive gibberish and innuendo stigmatised fatness and played into the hands of the ever-eager quack. A popular product of the period was Allan's Anti-Fat, which contained an extract of bladderwrack (seaweed). Many such products followed Pointing's advertising formula by providing informative 'anecdotes', such as this gem unearthed by Rance in the *Leeds Mercury* on 31 May 1879:

> *An exceedingly fat lady puffing like a steam engine, and clinging to the arm of a small wiry gentleman, whose face has become very red either from the unusual exercise or from the consciousness that a hundred eyes are looking at him with a ha! ha! in each pupil...*

Other slimming products, such as Figuroids, appealed to the more serious-minded patient, preferring science rather than personal insult to win over their customers. Advertisements for

Figuroids claimed that they had been: *'Discovered through an accident, while making Scientific investigations in the Laboratory'.*

George Dixon, who was managing director of the Figuroid Company, originated in Canada, where he had practised in Brockville, Ontario. His adverts for Figuroids stuck to the scientific approach, but aimed at bafflement rather than genuine information. According to Dixon, rival anti-fat products were ineffective because they sought to eliminate the fat within the body; however, no weight loss could occur until the fat was ejected from the body, by being made:

to pass out of the antipose cells into the little blood vessels, and it must there be oxidised and so converted into carbon-dioxide and water vapour, both of which are then eliminated readily from the body through the four great eliminating channels, the lungs, skin, kidneys and bowels.

All seemingly plausible, apart from the omission of precisely how Figuroids in any way aided this naturally occurring process.

As is clear, the door still remained open for quacks. In part, this was due to the Royal College of Physicians' continued rivalry with the pharmacists, in the form of the Society of Apothecaries, which had itself been granted permission to license pharmacists in 1815. (It had also been granted 'the power to license and regulate medical practitioners throughout England and Wales', though in fact this highly contentious power was rarely used.) On top of this, the College

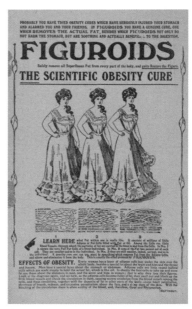

(Wellcome Library, London)

also faced rivalry from the new British Medical Association, which had been founded in 1832. And when the College instituted internal reforms during 1858–61, its new constitution stated:

The fellows and members are by the by-laws restricted from practising pharmacy, and from even indirectly supplying medicines to their patients: for, in England, it is held incompatible with the character of a physician that he should supply medicines to his patients, even though he does not make any direct charge for drugs.

Yet while institutions had been wary of over-zealous suppression of quacks, for fear of stoking up internecine rivalry, individuals had long carried out their own campaigns against quackery. It is worth mentioning a couple of these.

70

132

To make Plague Water

Sage, Sallendin, Rosemary, wormewood Muggworth,
dragons, Pimpernell, Scabious Egrimeny, Rosa-Solis,
Scordium, Sentery, Rew, Bittony Cardus Benedictus
Marygold flowers, of Each one handfull: Roots of Gentian
Tormentill, Elicompane, Angollico, Zedeary English Licorish
of each an ounce: beat roots and herbs in a a Stone Mortar
then Sleep um two dayes in a gallon of White-wine, and
one quart of Sack. Distill it in a rose-Still well pasted round
with rye-past, and the Reciever well stoped close with Browne
paper lett it runn on white sugar-candy two ounces to a
bottle: You may putt the first and Second running together
for that will make both good

133

To make haire growe where there is none

Take bees and burne um uppon a fire-shovell or some
such thing: then Boyle the ashes of the Bees in sallet oyle
then annoynt the place therewith where you would have
Haire growe, and in a short time you shall obtaine
your desire

DANIEL TURNER

Daniel Turner, a surgeon of considerable skill during the Georgian era, wielded arguments as deftly as he did his scalpel. Quacks were simply taken apart for their 'pitiful stock of knowledge'. Porter paraphrases his analysis:

> *They had mastered none of those approved continents of learning, from Greek and Latin to botany and anatomy, which every erudite practitioner required. Their books, bills, and patents bulged with grotesque blunders – of grammar, pharmacology, and diagnosis – which exposed them as arrant sociologists [charlatans].*

After all, what was a physician without Latin and Greek, without erudition and grammar, or even botany?

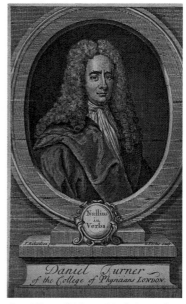

Daniel Turner, (Wellcome Library, London)

JAMES ADAIR, THE QUACK-FINDER GENERAL

Where Turner used a skilled scalpel, his contemporary James Makittrick Adair used a bludgeon. As early as the 1790s James Adair became the 'self-appointed Quack-Finder General'. And there is no doubt that Adair knew what he was talking about, for he himself had started in the medical profession as something of a quack. Having misspent his fortune in the taverns of Edinburgh, he quickly married a rich wife, whose fortune went the same way as his own. With no prior qualification, he then signed on as a surgeon's mate on a Royal Naval sloop bound for the West Indies. Here he took up an appointment as manager of a sugar plantation, where he was horrified at the treatment of the black slaves. He treated these unfortunates with deep compassion, but a seemingly inborn contrariness then caused him to write a pamphlet entitled *Unanswerable Arguments against the Abolition of the Slave Trade.* At the same time, he also 'began to study the medical profession'. However, it was only several years later – after he took a tour of the United States, where he too met Benjamin Franklin – that he returned to England and began to study medicine in an orthodox manner.

Later, Adair would take up practice in Bath, where he became involved in all manner of disputes with his fellow physicians. One assessment has it that: 'He was naturally querulous, hot, and irascible, and his disposition had been soured by disappointments in domestic life.' The physicians of Bath proved tough enemies, but the fashionable quacks of Bath (and elsewhere) were no match for Adair's thundering rage, which was nonetheless capable of penetrating argument. Perhaps his most notable enemy was Thomas Godbold, who had gained entry to high society and an income of £10,000 a year from his Vegetable Balsam. This he claimed could cure both asthma and consumption, while in Adair's view 'anyone but a blithering idiot knew these were utterly diverse disorders requiring clean contrary therapeutics'. Adair may have been the scourge of quacks, but his unassuageable anger soon caused him to widen his target. In 1787 he would write:

> *In all departments of life quackery prevails. Hence we have Imperial quacks (as the present Emperor has experienced to his cost); legislative quacks, who tamper with political constitutions which they do not understand; philosophical, ethical, critical and religious quacks.*

The Emperor he refers to is the Habsburg Emperor Joseph II, patron of Mozart, whose health had been ruined by the misdiagnoses of the imperial physicians and who would die three years later. Adair would continue on his cantankerous way for another twelve years, on one notable occasion his apoplectic behaviour causing him to be confined to Winchester jail. According to a historical source: 'He became hypochondriacal and died at Harrogate in 1802'.

JOHN ST JOHN LONG

The fame, fortune and public adulation attained by some quacks in the early 19th century is evident in the case of John St John Long who was referred to in The Lancet as 'the King of Humbugs'. Born in Newcastle, County Limerick in 1798, Long studied art at the Dublin Academy before moving to London in 1822. He spent a few years working as an artist and his paintings were exhibited at the Society of British Artists and the British Institution in 1824–25.

Life as an artist did not pay well and Long decided to practise medicine. Despite having no medical training or qualifications – just a knowledge of anatomy acquired from his study of art – he built up a very successful practice in Harley Street, promoting a cure for a number of diseases including gout and consumption. Long had rich and powerful patients and was particularly admired by women. He was secretive about his methods and asked his patients to sign a book to say that they would not pass on details of the treatment they received although it was known to involve the inhalation of vapours or rubbing his unique lotion into the back, shoulders or chest. One patient who was treated said that it involved producing a wound on the back, rubbing in a lotion every day for five to ten days and then covering the weeping wound with cabbage leaves.

In 1830 Long was asked by Mrs Cashin to treat her 16-year-old daughter, Ellen, who had consumption. Although he saw Ellen, Long told her mother that he could not cure her. Mrs Cashin became concerned that her other daughter, 24-year-old Catherine, might suffer the same fate as her sister and asked Long to use his methods to prevent her from getting the disease. Long agreed. The treatment did not go well and the wound on Catherine's back increased in size over the following days and it was not long before she was in great agony and unable to hold down food or drink. Long remained unconcerned, telling the family that her back was in the state he expected it to be and that she would recover in a few days. In desperation, the family called in the eminent surgeon Benjamin Brodie but unfortunately Catherine died the following day.

A coroner's inquest returned a verdict of manslaughter and Long was sent for trial at the Old Bailey. Several medical witnesses told both the inquest and the trial that they could not imagine how Long's treatment could cure consumption. They had no doubt that the treatment had caused Catherine's death. The trial heard:

"The state of the back appeared as if produced by a scorching heat; if a piece of red hot iron nearly the size of a crown of a hat had been applied for about a quarter of an hour, it would have produced a similar appearance. The skin was completely destroyed."

Despite evidence from more than 60 patients that the treatment was effective Long was convicted of manslaughter. He was fined £250, which he paid immediately and then went on to continue to practise as before.

Less than four months later in February 1831, Long was at the Old Bailey again. This time he was accused of the manslaughter of Mrs Colin Campbell Lloyd who had died in similar circumstances to Catherine Cashin. To the delight of his supporters as well as the women who sat in the dock with him, but to the great dismay of the medical profession, he was acquitted.

Long died just three years later, not after failing to use his own remedy to treat his supposed consumption but following a riding accident and a ruptured blood vessel caused by a cough. His secret remedy which had been bought for £10,000 was found to contain turpentine, vinegar and egg-yolk.

FOLLOWING PAGE: John St John Long at the Old Bailey

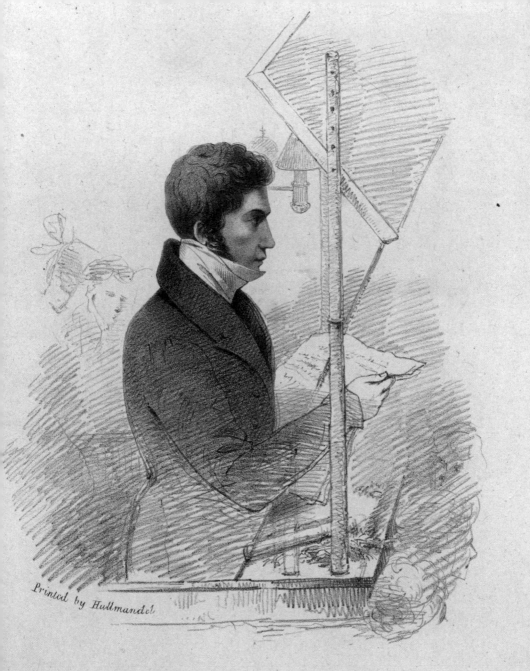

Printed by Hullmandel

Mr JOHN St JOHN LONG.

as he appeared on his Defence at the Old Bailey 19 Feby. 1831.

DRAWN FROM LIFE. AND ON STONE BY J. FAHEY.

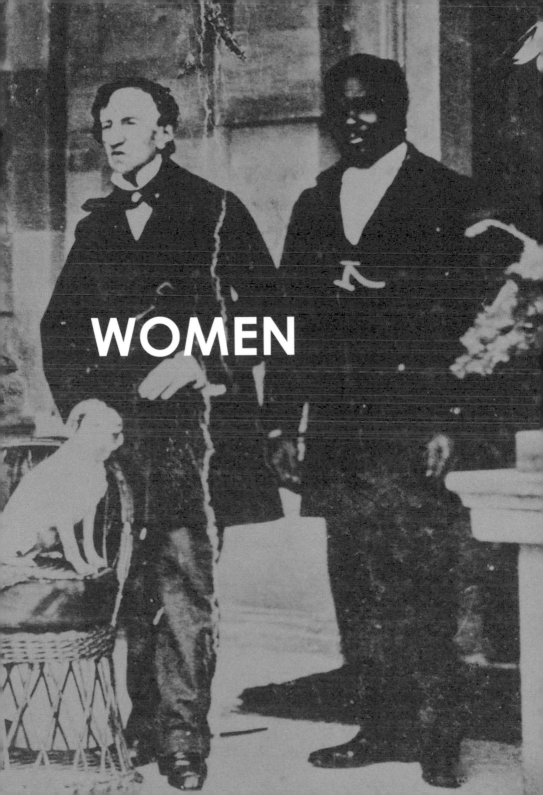

JAMES BARRY

The ensuing generation would see perhaps the most successful medical fraud of them all in the form of Dr James Miranda Stuart Barry, who rose to become the senior Inspector-General in the British Army. The first clue to the fraud lies in the name Miranda, although this was said to have been taken from the exiled Latin American general, Francisco de Miranda, who became an early mentor. Dr James Barry was in fact born Miranda Stuart 'around 1795' and she was probably the scion of a Scottish aristocratic family. Little is known of her early life, but by the time she appeared with the enveloping masculine name James Barry and joined the army as a hospital assistant, she had already gained medical qualifications at Edinburgh University. Now permanently posing as a male, 1816 saw her posted as an assistant surgeon to the Cape of Good Hope Colony, at the remote tip of Africa. At the time, this was a frontier port on the edge of the Empire and existence was primitive. Barry quickly attracted attention, as much for her independent and wilful manner as for her compassion for her patients – who included prostitutes, sailors and black slaves. Although Barry went to great lengths to exhibit her manliness, becoming 'a skilled marksman, drinking and telling stories in the mess with the men', her beardless face, 'reddish hair and high cheekbones' led one of her more perceptive companions to remark: 'There was a certain effeminacy in his manner which he was always striving to overcome.' Though this same companion couldn't help but remark that 'his style of conversation was greatly superior to that one usually heard at a mess table in those days'.

One of Barry's duties was to act as personal physician to the Governor of the Cape Colony, the maverick aristocrat Lord Charles Somerset, who shared Barry's enlightened attitude towards the black slaves. When Somerset was struck down with cholera, it was Barry who saved his life. She revealed to him her secret and they fell in love. Lady Somerset soon became aghast at the rumours of her husband's homosexual entanglement and in London a bishop called for a commission to be set up to investigate the matter. Barry was exonerated, but by then Lord Somerset had returned to England.

Through skill, dedication and social ability, Barry rose quickly through the ranks. By the outbreak of the Crimean War, she had become an Inspector General, in which capacity she inspected the hospital at Scutari run by Florence Nightingale, becoming outraged at its atrocious and unhygienic conditions. Nightingale was a determined woman, but would later describe how she was forced to endure the worst 'scolding' in her entire life. It was this which led Nightingale to understand the fundamental need for hygiene.

Barry would die in 1865, at around the age of seventy. She would take her secret to her death but not to her grave. The results of her autopsy caused a huge scandal in Victorian England.

PREVIOUS PAGE: James Barry with dog and servant (Army Medical Services Muniment Collection in care of the Wellcome Library)

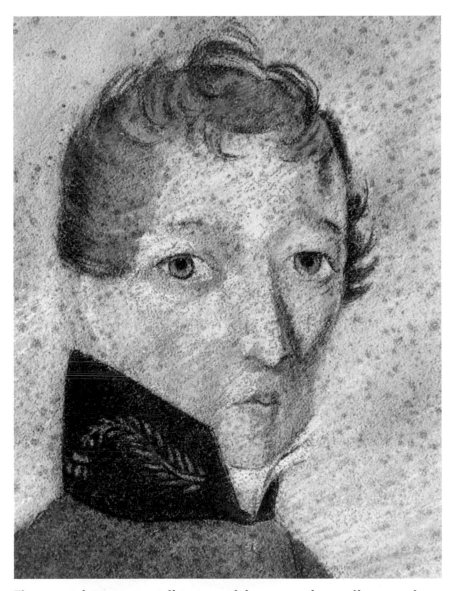

The ensuing generation would see perhaps the most successful medical fraud of them all in the form of Dr James Miranda Stuart Barry, who rose to become the senior Inspector-General in the British Army.

(Army Medical Services Muniment Collection in care of the Wellcome Library)

The topic of a woman fraudulently posing as a male doctor brings us into the modern era. Barry may have been a fraud, but she was definitely no quack. But why was a woman unable to enter the medical profession, except as a fraud in disguise? Other 'frauds' seeking a way around this discrimination were already appearing on the scene. In the words of Sir Christopher Booth, in his contribution to a history of the Royal College of Physicians:

> *The Medical Act of 1858 set up the General Medical Council as a self-regulatory body to implement and monitor standards of training. There were no restrictions in this Act on allowing women to present themselves for assessment and registration. It was largely the individual universities and medical schools in the UK who barred women from entry and training and thus* de facto *women were excluded from presenting themselves to the licensing bodies including the Royal College of Physicians.*

ELIZABETH BLACKWELL

One woman who found a way around this Catch-22 was Elizabeth Blackwell, who was born in Bristol in 1821. When she was just eleven, her family emigrated to America where Blackwell eventually became a school teacher. Although she had a certain distaste for bodily functions, she took up studying medicine during the holidays 'to dissuade a persistent suitor, and also to register her outrage over the unequal

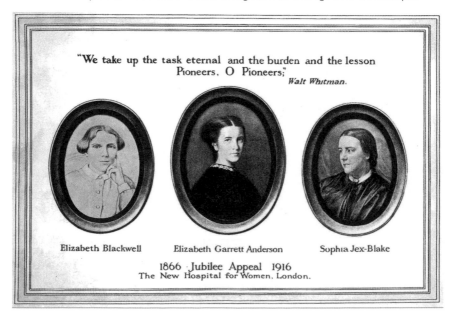

"We take up the task eternal and the burden and the lesson Pioneers, O Pioneers."
Walt Whitman.

Elizabeth Blackwell   Elizabeth Garrett Anderson   Sophia Jex-Blake

1866 Jubilee Appeal 1916
The New Hospital for Women, London.

ABOVE: (Wellcome Library, London)
PREVIOUS PAGE: Six vignettes of self-help hydrotherapy (Wellcome Library, London)

treatment of women'. Blackwell was a determined woman, but when she applied to study medicine in Philadelphia she was turned down by all four of the local medical schools. This made her even more determined, so she cast further afield and applied to the Geneva Medical School in upstate New York.

These were stormy times in American universities and the students at Geneva were in a state of open rebellion against the university authorities. In a gesture intended to heal the breach, the authorities handed over the decision concerning Blackwell's entry to the all-male student body. However, in a move intended to get back at the authorities, the students accepted Blackwell 'as a practical joke'. Blackwell determined to take this 'practical joke' seriously and turned up to study. Despite social ostracism throughout the community, who judged her to be either 'mad or bad', she duly graduated top of her year. Now that she had a degree she travelled briefly to England, but soon went back to America. In 1869 she returned permanently to Britain and established the London School of Medicine for Women. Were all the graduates of this school to be rejected as quacks and frauds? They might have been, but for the determination of the first woman to qualify as a doctor in England.

ELIZABETH GARRETT ANDERSON

The woman now known as Elizabeth Garrett Anderson was born in Whitechapel in 1836, where her father had been a pawnbroker. Business flourished in this poor district and Elizabeth was sent to a private school. On leaving, she encountered the newly qualified Elizabeth Blackwell on her early visit to England. Anderson was inspired to become a doctor. In 1865 she obtained a diploma from the Society of Apothecaries. This technically allowed her to enrol on the medical register, even though she was not a qualified doctor. She then crossed to Paris, where she took a medical degree. On her return, the Royal College of Physicians refused her the chance of a licence, on the grounds that its by-laws did not allow women to sit their exams. She then enrolled at the British Medical Association, who later claimed that her enrolment was due to 'a bureaucratic error'. But by now it was too late, as all agreed, and in 1876 the Gurney Act was passed removing all restriction from the medical profession on grounds of sex. The Royal College of Physicians fought a rearguard action, with one aged fellow suggesting 'that if girls were encouraged to use their brains the excitement caused thereby would produce insanity'. But by the turn of the century even the College had decided to throw in the towel. Women doctors were no longer quacks or frauds *by definition*.

The nineteenth and twentieth centuries would witness a sea change in the nature of quackery. Just as politicians, philosophers and even individual scientists gave birth to collective movements (Darwinism, Marxism, atomism, to name but a few), so quackery produced its own ideologies. And like their other social counterparts, many of these remain controversial to this day.

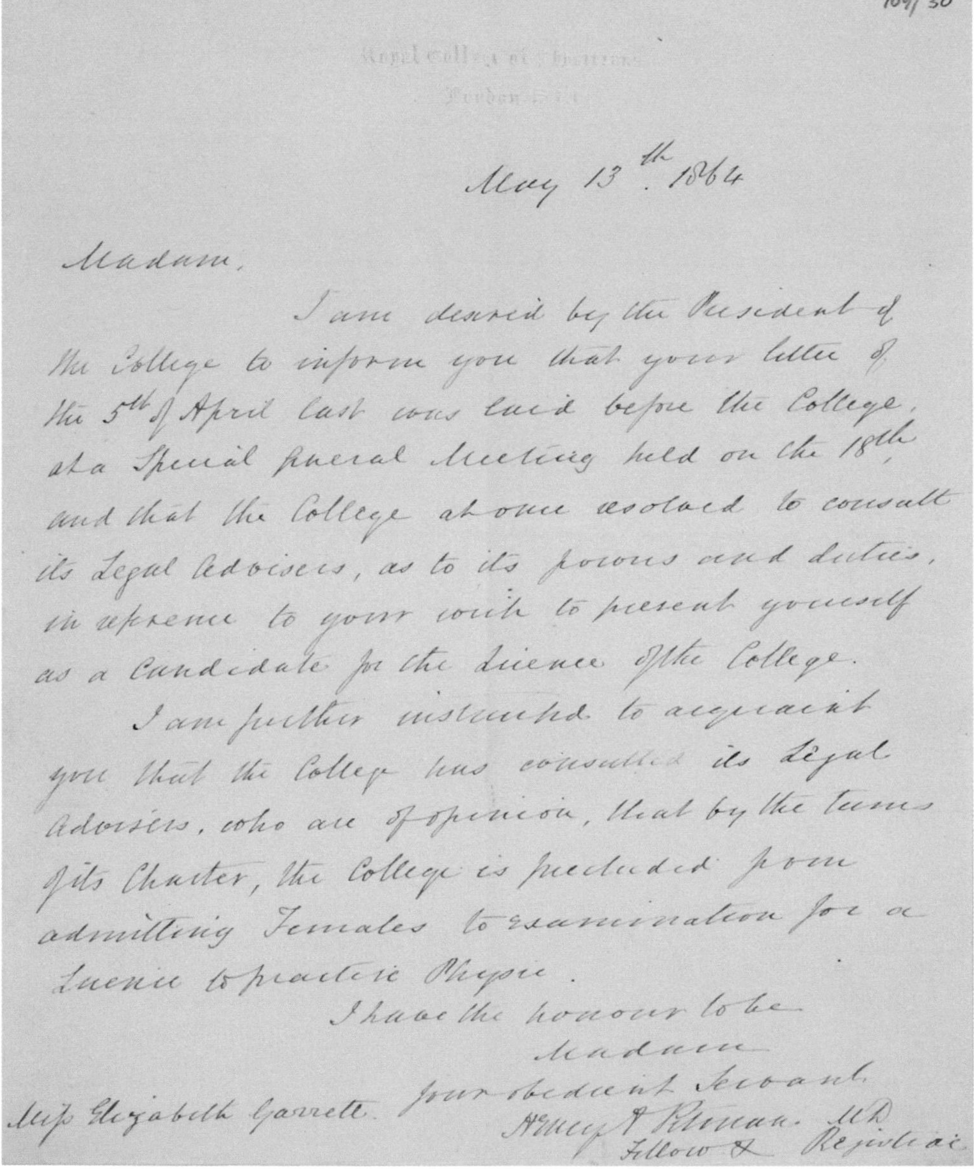

109/30

Royal College of Physicians
London S.W.

May 13th 1864

Madam,

I am desired by the President of
the College to inform you that your letter of
the 5th of April last was laid before the College,
at a Special General Meeting held on the 18th,
and that the College at once resolved to consult
its Legal Advisers, as to its powers and duties,
in reference to your wish to present yourself
as a Candidate for the Licence of the College.

I am further instructed to acquaint
you that the College has consulted its Legal
Advisers, who are of opinion, that by the terms
of its Charter, the College is precluded from
admitting Females to examination for a
Licence to practise Physic.

I have the honour to be
Madam
your obedient Servant
Henry & Pitman. MD
Fellow & Registrar

Miss Elizabeth Garrett.

Letters to and from Elizabeth Garrett in the RCP collections

Oct 19/95
ack⁴ + thanks

2th Ans⁴ reporting
Oct. Reso⁴ⁿ of College declining
to grant the prayer of the Petition

London School of Medicine for Women,
30, Handel Street,
Brunswick Square, W.C.

Oct 17ᵗʰ 1895

Sir

I have now the honour of placing in your hands a list of the various Universities & Examining bodies which admit women to their medical examinations, degrees or diplomas, together with copies of the Enabling Act generally known as the 'Russell Gurney Act.'

I am, Sir
Yours obediently
E Garrett Anderson
Dean of the London School of
Medicine for Women

To the Registrar of the Royal
College of Physicians

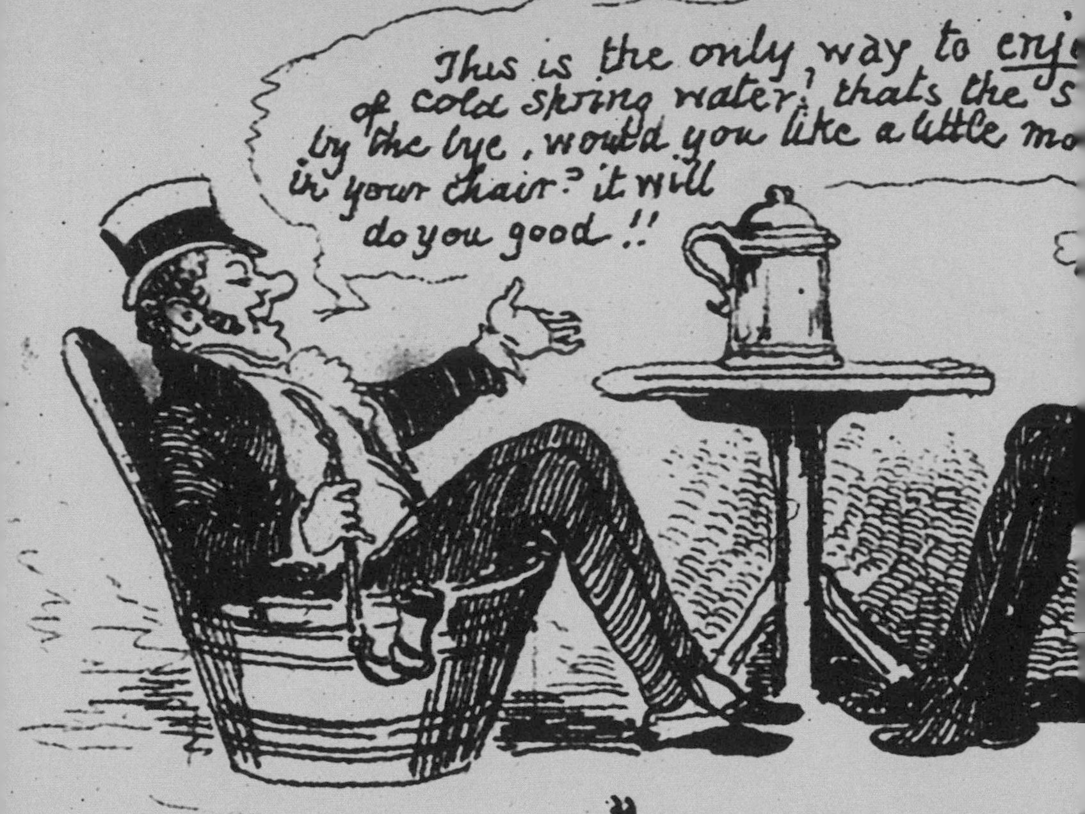

A "COOL TANKARD

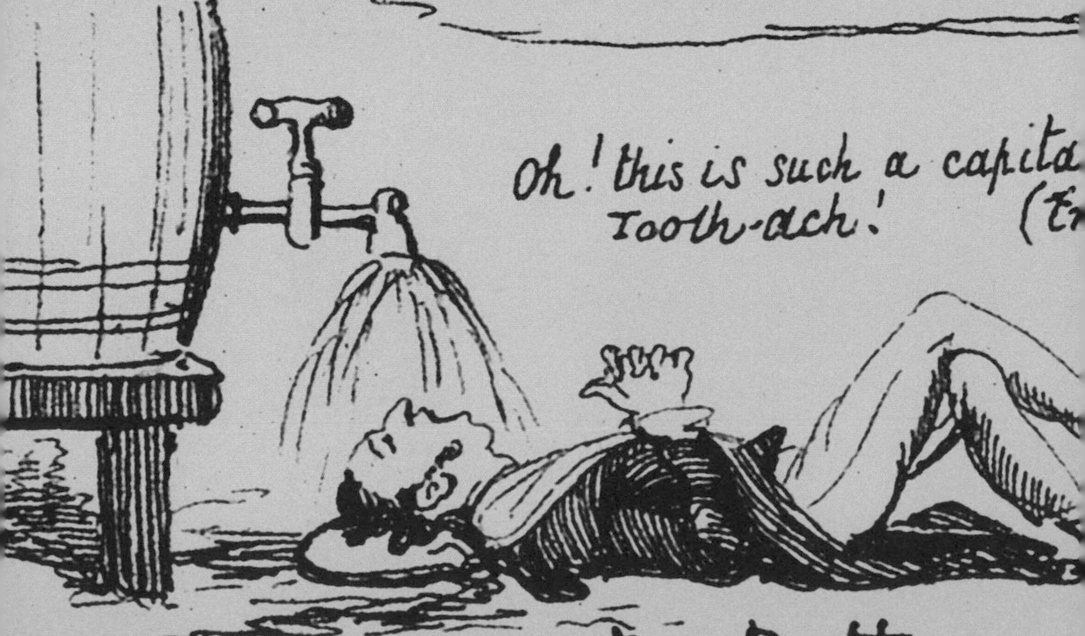

The Water Butt

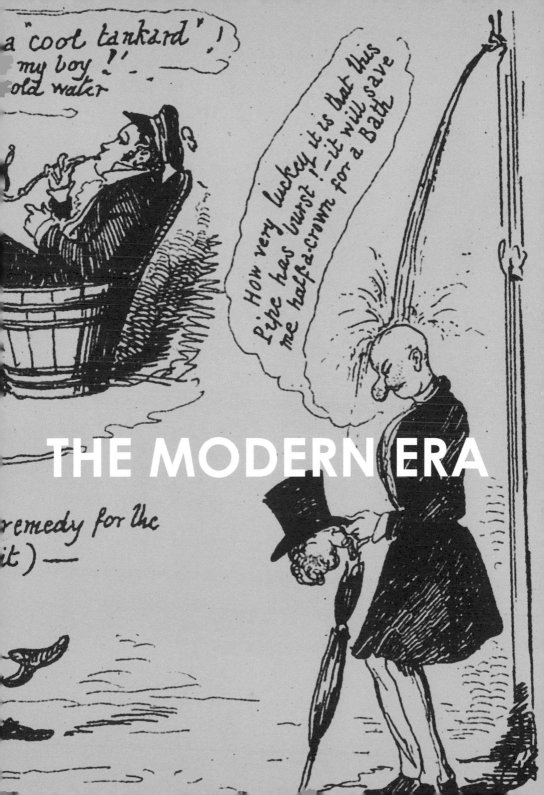

HYDROTHERAPY

The idea of the 'water cure' would revive long-forgotten spas all over Europe. Towns from Baden-Baden to Bath, from Karlsbad to Vichy, became fashionable resorts, where high society (and their attendant 'curers', dietary counsellors, 'healers' and the like) came to take the waters of the local spa. These usually gushed from a hot spring producing more or less sulphurous, malodorous, 'radioactive' or foul-tasting water. Such waters could be sprinkled, bathed in, drunk, endured as steam or ice, or used in other ingenious methods – all said to grant restorative powers to the jaded constitution.

The therapeutic powers of water had been extolled since ancient times, going as far back as ancient Egypt. These powers underwent a general revival around the turn of the nineteenth century, when such practices acquired a scientific nomenclature in the form of 'hydrotherapy', 'balneotherapy' and such. The craze for 'water cures' originated in Germany and Austria under such figures as Vincenz Priessnitz, the 'nature prophet', who introduced naturopathic medicine. This was (and is) a blanket term for a whole range of 'holistic medicines' with more or less dubious practices. Though lacking in scientific rigour, few of these practices are actually dangerous, apart from opposition to inoculation and claims to cure cancer. Priessnitz's 'water cure' methods gained great credence in Germany with their 'no pain, no gain' principle. According to Porter:

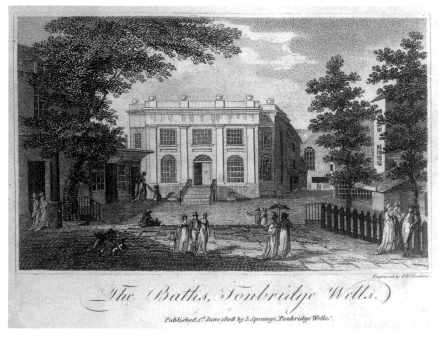

The Baths, Tonbridge Wells.

Published 1st June 1808 by I. Sprange, Tonbridge Wells.

ABOVE: (Wellcome Library, London)
OPPOSITE: A man taking a shower as part of a hydrotherapeutic cure (Wellcome Library, London)

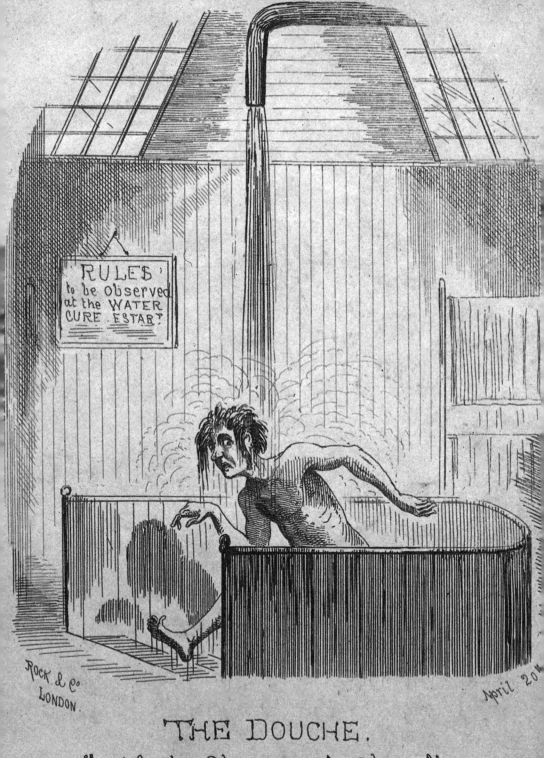

THE DOUCHE.

"Oh! Oh! Oh! Oh!"

The cold douche was the **coup de grâce:** *icy water was discharged over patients from a height of twenty feet. These were spartan methods, but they worked well on an overfed, overdrugged and stressed-out generation.*

And this was the point. Spas stressed healthy living and after a week or two away from customary over-indulgence, many returned home feeling 'cured'. In England, the lack of emphasis on the 'pain' element attracted all manner of distinguished, and otherwise rational, patients from Thomas Carlyle to Alfred Lord Tennyson, and even Charles Darwin, who was a great believer in regularly taking the waters. But it was the very success of the spas which contributed to their decline. As they became more fashionable, they increasingly hosted more fashionable pursuits. With the introduction of casinos, society balls and gourmet restaurants, it was not long before the likes of Dostoyevsky were gambling away their fortune in manic fashion and Edward VII was riding his carriage along the local river bed in the early hours. Such figures, and their emulators, were seldom attracted to therapeutic baths or icy waterfalls, and the fashionable crowd moved on to other such hot and cold spots as Monte Carlo and Gstaad.

Many such collective crazes of modern quackery originated abroad, before taking root more or less successfully in England.

Many such collective crazes of modern quackery originated abroad, before taking root more or less successfully in England. The main foreign source of such ideas has been America. Where medicine was concerned, this was undeniably the 'land of the free'. Following the Declaration of Independence in 1776, the pharmaceutical scene was left almost entirely devoid of regulatory control. While snake oil salesmen flourished in the Wild West, other more dangerous concoctions and drugs were freely available at pharmacists throughout the land. Opium-based medicines with names such as 'Bracer' and 'Soothing Syrup' became popular over-the-counter items. Indeed, the original 1885 Coca-Cola actually contained cocaine. Not until 1929 (*sic!*) did Coke become entirely coke-free. As for the more exotic soothing syrups and such, these were not eliminated until the Pure Food and Drug Act of 1906 (which seemingly overlooked Coca-Cola). When Coca-Cola crossed the Atlantic and became popular in Britain in the first decades of the twentieth century it could hardly be described as a fraud (its very name proclaimed its magic ingredient) and it would thus be difficult to stigmatise its effects as quackery. On the other hand, cocaine was a known narcotic.[8] This meant that Coca-Cola was hardly the health-giving drink it claimed to be – despite this, early slogans in Britain proclaimed it as 'the great temperance beverage' and 'pure as sunlight'.

JOHN HARVEY KELLOGG

Ironically, another popular product that crossed the Atlantic at this time, which was wholly devoid of narcotic substances, was in fact created by an undeniable quack. This was John Harvey Kellogg, who presided over a sanitarium in Battle Creek, Michigan. Although qualified as an orthodox doctor, he preferred to employ an alternative 'holistic' approach at his sanitarium. His treatment emphasised exercise, vegetarianism and enemas. On the other hand, he went out of his way to discourage all surgery, which was liable to cause an 'imbalance' in the body. Worse still were his recommendations with regard to sexuality. Despite being against surgery, he prescribed circumcision as a cure for masturbation. Paradoxically, he also prescribed sewing up the foreskin to prevent this practice, while for women he directed the application of carbolic acid to the clitoris. This was also the man, who together with his brother William Keith Kellogg, invented cornflakes.

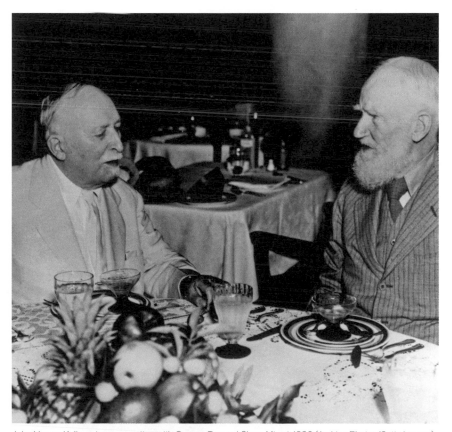

John Harvey Kellogg in conversation with George Bernard Shaw, Miami 1936 (Archive Photos/Getty Images)

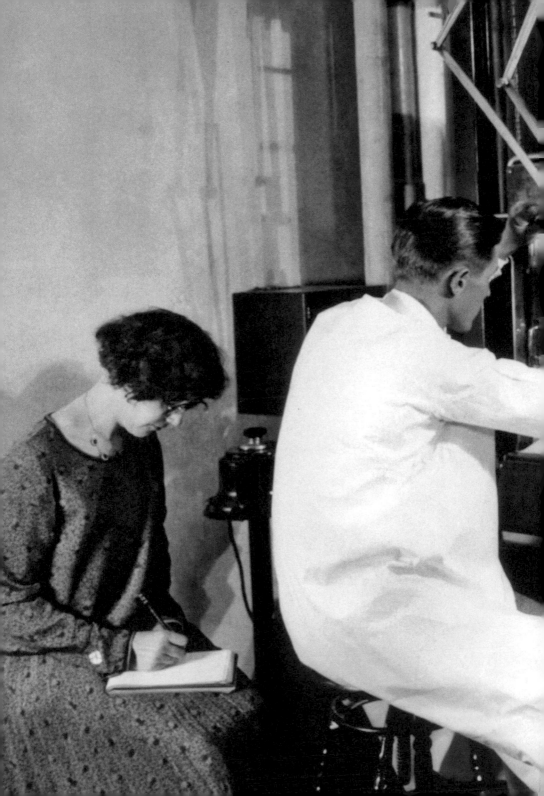

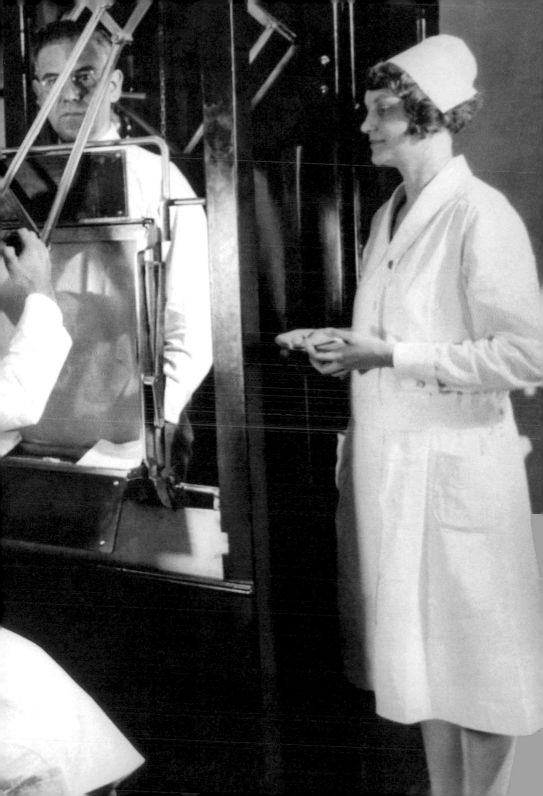

NORMAN HAIRE

Other popular but controversial practices which flourished in the twentieth century were associated with the field of sexology. As ever, in the tradition of James Graham and his Grand Celestial Bed, this subject attracted all manner of weird practitioners and wonderful treatments. A number of these were genuinely beneficial – as in the case of the German Magnus Hirschfeld and his Institute for Sexual Research in Berlin. This did much to promote the cause and understanding of homosexuality, even if a veil is best drawn over some of its more 'naturopathic' methods. Hirschfeld's work was introduced to Britain by the writers Christopher Isherwood and W. H. Auden.

A less respectable practitioner in this field was Norman Haire, who would become associated with all manner of writers, celebrities and intellectuals – from H. G. Wells to Charles Laughton, as well as W. B. Yeats, who even went so far as to undergo his so-called 'Steinach treatment for rejuvenation'. In fact, this was no more than a vasectomy, yet according to Haire's claims his treatment not only revitalised the

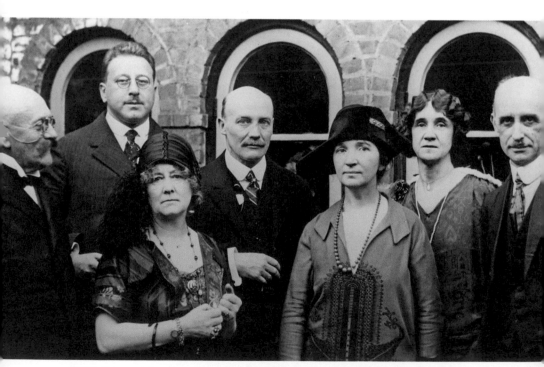

ABOVE: Representatives at a Birth Control Conference (from left) Georges Vacher deLapouge, Norman Haire, Thit Jensen, Charles Vickery, C.V. Drysdale, Juliet Barrett Rublee and Gabriel Hardy outside Mrs Rublee's house in New York. (General Photographic Agency/Getty Images)
PREVIOUS PAGE: A physician doing a fluoroscope examination at John Harvey Kellogg's Battlecreek sanatorium, Michigan, c. 1928 (Underwood Archives/Getty Images)

sex life of his ageing patients, but also reversed the effects of senility. (Women could have their ovaries 'irradiated' with similar effect.) In the wake of Freud and his new psychoanalysis, sex was very much the topic of the moment, with quack sexologists offering such operations as 'monkey gland treatment', the engraftment of goats' testicles and the like.

Norman Haire was born in Australia of Jewish parents, and qualified in medicine in Sydney. Upon his arrival in London in 1918 he quickly transformed himself from being an unknown doctor with a colonial background into a highly successful Harley Street gynaecologist, complete with Rolls-Royce and country mansion. According to his biography: 'He was a feeling, thinking and doing man, equal parts hedonist and humanist; a tall, fat and flamboyant rationalist who was secretly homosexual.' This last secret led him to visit Hirschfeld's Institute in Berlin in 1923, after which he devoted more of his energies to sexology. His 'rejuvenation operation', pioneered by the later discredited Eugen Steinach in Vienna, became a fad, and Haire modestly claimed to have performed this on 'rather less than 200' artists, writers, celebrities and intellectuals. Despite its lack of scientific basis, Haire's operation certainly appeared to 'work' – largely through psychosomatic effects, autosuggestion or the unwillingness of patients to publicly admit their continuing impotence and decrepitude. Haire's treatment might have been fraudulent, but any who doubt its transformative effects need only study the case of W. B. Yeats, on whom Haire operated in 1934 when the poet was aged sixty-nine. Consequently, during the last four years of his life Yeats experienced what he called his 'second puberty', which caused him to produce a burst of vigorous and inspired late poems, at the same time launching himself into an enthusiastic and chaotic love life. Charlatans they may be, but there is no denying that quacks can sometimes perform a service – if only to literature, rather than marital relations.

Charlatans they may be, but there is no denying that quacks can sometimes perform a service – if only to literature, rather than marital relations.

CONTEMPORARY QUACKERY

All this brings us to the present day, which boasts quacks, frauds and charlatans of all the types which have characterised the previous developments of this human endeavour, though in modern guise. The common shouting quacks of old have now abandoned the street for the TV studio and the internet, eschewing such outdated props as performing moneys and snakes in favour of beaming actors performing as satisfied patients. Modern charlatans who descend from the more enlightened era of quackery now tend to practise their art as 'healers' (faith or otherwise), purveyors of miracle diets, and of course sexologists, often presiding over their own clinic or health resort. Then of course there are those who aspire to the third stage, preaching more serious medical 'philosophies', scientific movements, or simply peddling their wares (ideological or pharmaceutical) on a global scale, especially in third world countries.

One aspect of all but the most amateurish of these contemporary quacks or multinational frauds is their willingness to resort to the law to 'protect their good name'. Hence my somewhat anonymous treatment of this most recent evolution of quackery, whose particular practitioners will surely spring to the mind of the informed reader. Alas, any further prompting on this matter would only involve the Royal College of Physicians (and myself) in tedious and costly litigation…

And so what are the lessons to be learned from all this? Quacks, frauds and charlatans remain as pervasive as ever. But the forces ranging against them have also adapted to the modern world. As patients have become more educated they have tended to become less susceptible to more modern forms of medical deception. Yet problems remain: the internet abounds in quacks describing symptoms and recommending their own patent cures – and every day such con-men become ever more pervasive. People stricken with illnesses (real or imagined) will always crave reassurance almost as much as they long to be cured. Not for nothing has confidence trickery sometimes been known as the world's second-oldest profession. And as such, quacks, frauds and charlatans will doubtless always remain a flourishing offshoot of the genuine practice of medicine.

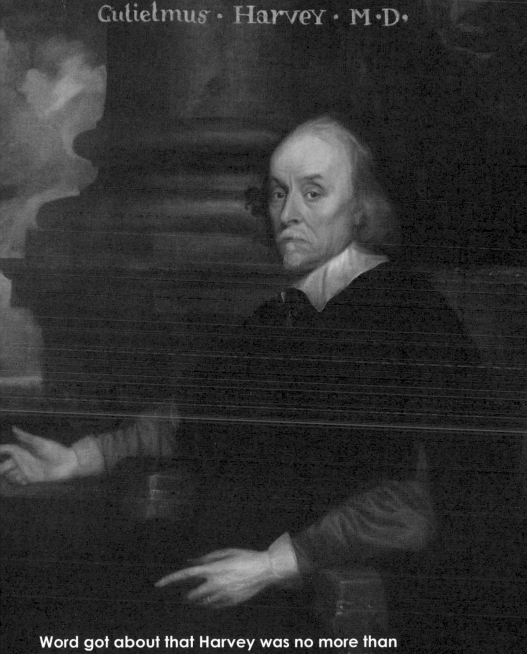

Gulielmus · Harvey · M·D·

Word got about that Harvey was no more than
a quack and the conservative element in the
Royal College of Physicians began referring to
him as 'Harvey the circulator' – a double-edged
epithet (*circulator* is Latin for quack).

SELECT BIBLIOGRAPHY

Sir George Clark, *A History of the Royal College of Physicians,* 4 volumes (Oxford 1964 *et seq.*)

Geoffrey Davenport (ed.), *The Royal College of Physicians and its Collections* (London 2001)

Hempel S. 'John St John Long: quackery and manslaughter', *The Lancet* 3 May 2014; 383:1540–1

Hutt, M. Long, 'John St John (1798–1834)', Oxford dictionary of national biography, Oxford University Press, 2004 [http://www.oxforddnb.com/view/article/16971, accessed 22 October 2015]

Roy Porter, *Quacks* (London 1989)

Roy Porter, *The Greatest Benefit to Mankind* (London 1999)

Caroline Rance, *The Quack Doctor,* (Stroud 2013)

Extraordinary inquest – Mr St John Long, *The Spectator*, 28 August 1830, 650–653

Paul Strathern, *A Brief History of Medicine* (London 2005)

C. J. S. Thompson, *The Quacks of Old London* (London 1928)

ENDNOTES

1. Dr Johnson would increasingly suffer from this disease for the remaining seventy-two years of his life. He would also include the word 'quack' in his first dictionary, as 'a boastful pretender to arts which he does not understand'.

2. The actual term snake oil salesman, in its modern usage, originated in the American West during the era of pioneers and cowboys in the early nineteenth century. However, for several centuries prior to this quacks selling 'snake oil' as a panacea were prevalent in Europe. Authentic European snake oil, such as that sold in London during the early days of the Royal College of Physicians, was usually prepared from vipers. Other less scrupulous preparations might include such ingredients as camphor, pepper or turpentine. Both the 'authentic' and the lesser elixirs were equally devoid of curative powers. To this day, genuine snake oils can be purchased in the Far East, but their powers match those of the original product.

3. George I had two German mistresses of such unprepossessing appearance that they became known as 'The Maypole and The Elephant'. Presumably 'Crazy Sally' was mistaken for the latter.

4. i.e. with just his head protruding from the earth.

5. At the grand old age of fifty-two, Sydenham would finally remedy this omission by taking an MD at Cambridge. According to an official historian of the Royal College of Physicians: 'Sydenham was not a Fellow…but such was his contribution to medicine…that he was greatly esteemed by the Fellows of the College.'

6. Such a name was not quite so comic as it might appear. This was the time when Thomas Crapper and his colleagues were developing the flush toilet for the new bourgeois market. As one modern commentator has seen fit to point out: 'These were the Bill Gates and Steve Jobs of their day.'

7. Ward's fortune and fame had long since scotched any doubting rumours concerning his products. Such side-effects of quackery would soon be seen in fields far beyond medicine, where they continue to this day. Founders of billion-dollar investment schemes (e.g. Bernard Madoff), as well as over-leveraged newspaper proprietors (e.g. Robert Maxwell) relied for their success upon just this quack quality.

8. In the late nineteeth century, Sir Arthur Conan Doyle famously launched a vain attempt to undermine the popularity of his creation Sherlock Holmes by portraying him as a habitual user of cocaine.

FOLLOWING PAGES: James Gillray's 'Metallic – Tractors' and George Cruickshank's 'The Cholic' and 'The Head ache'

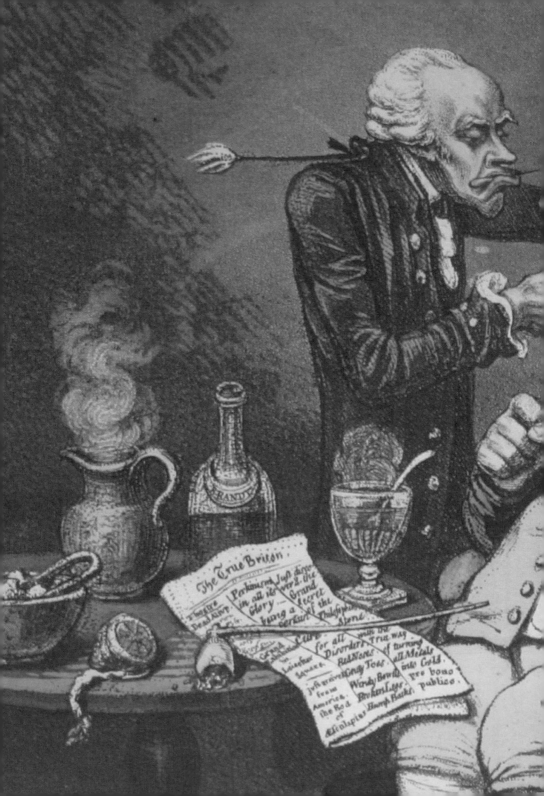

The True Briton

Positive
Reading

Parkinson just disposed
in all its over 2 the
glory   Grand
                having a secret
                certain of the
                       Philosophers
                       Stone

Grand Cure   for all   with the
in Leicester   Square   Bad Noses   of turning
                        Only Toes   all Metals
just arrived   Wind y Bowls   into Gold
from   Windy Bowels
America   Broken Legs   pro bono
the Rod of   publico.
Æsculapius   Hump Backs

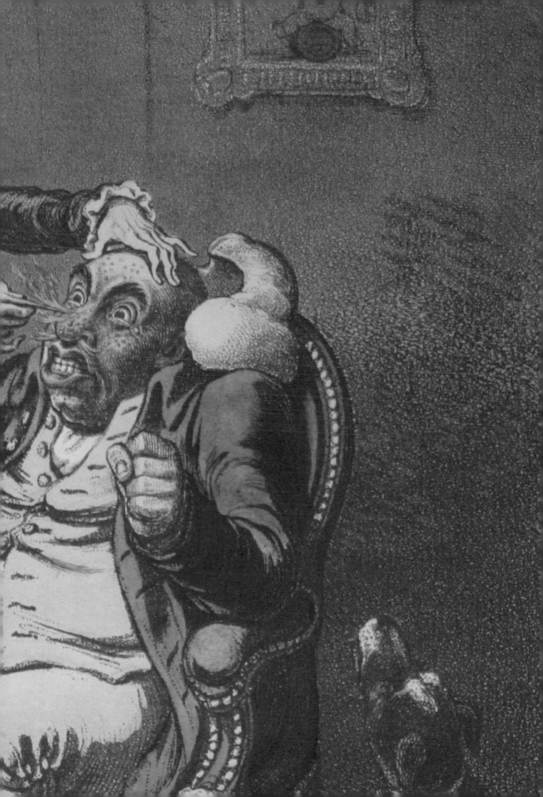

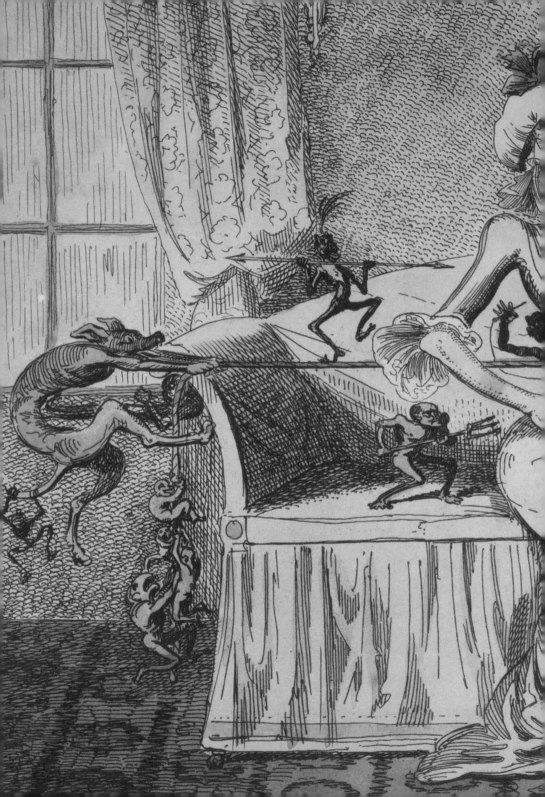

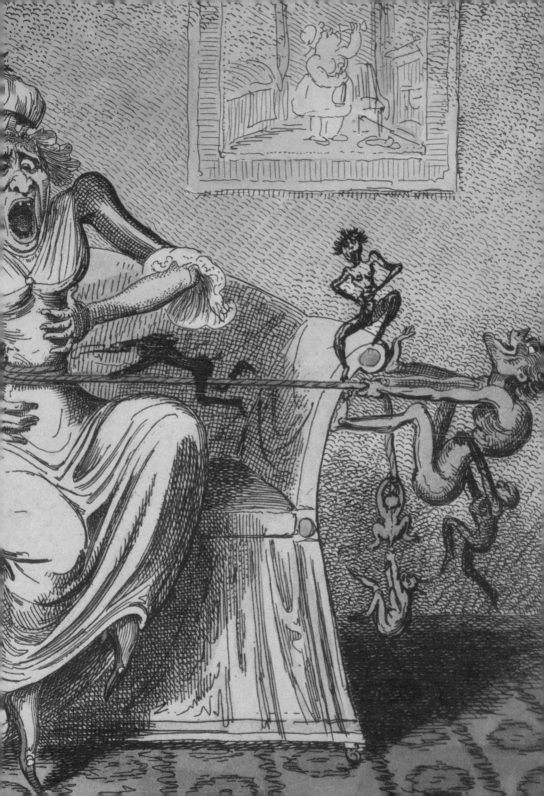

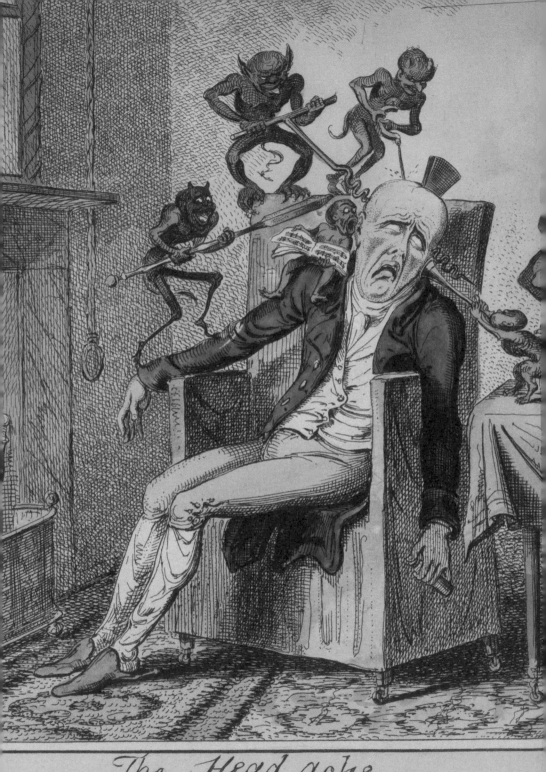

The Head ache